Selling Teaching Hospitals and Practice Plans

Also by the Author

Arrhythmias

Mergers of Teaching Hospitals in Boston, New York, and Northern California

Governance of Teaching Hospitals: Turmoil at Penn and Hopkins

Specialty Care in the Era of Managed Care: Cleveland Clinic versus University Hospitals of Cleveland

You and Your Arrhythmia: A Guide to Cardiac Arrhythmias for Patients and Families

Selling Teaching Hospitals and Practice Plans

George Washington and
Georgetown Universities

John A. Kastor, M.D.
Professor, Department of Medicine
University of Maryland School of Medicine
Baltimore, Maryland

The Johns Hopkins University Press
Baltimore

The Johns Hopkins University Press
2715 North Charles Street
Baltimore, Maryland 21218-4363
www.press.jhu.edu

Library of Congress Cataloging-in-Publication Data

Kastor, John A.
  Selling teaching hospitals and practice plans : George
Washington and Georgetown Universities / John A. Kastor.
    p. ; cm.
  Includes bibliographical references and index.
  ISBN-13: 978-0-8018-8811-3 (hardcover : alk. paper)
  ISBN-10: 0-8018-8811-5 (hardcover : alk. paper)
  1. Teaching hospitals—Washington (D.C.)—Administration.
2. Teaching hospitals—Washington (D.C.)—Finance. 3. Academic
medical centers—Washington (D.C.)—Administration.
4. Hospitals—Ownership—Washington (D.C.) 5. George
Washington University. Medical Center. 6. Georgetown
University. Medical Center. I. Title.
  [DNLM: 1. George Washington University. 2. Georgetown
University. 3. Academic Medical Centers—organization &
administration—District of Columbia. 4. Financial
Management—District of Columbia. 5. Hospital Restructuring—
District of Columbia. 6. Practice Management—District of
Columbia. WX 27 AD6 K19s 2008]
  RA975.T43K376 2008
  362.1109753—dc22   2007038399

A catalog record for this book is available from the British Library.

Special discounts are available for bulk purchases of this book. For
more information, please contact Special Sales at 410-516-6936 or
specialsales@press.jhu.edu.

The Johns Hopkins University Press uses environmentally
friendly book materials, including recycled text paper that is
composed of at least 30 percent post-consumer waste, whenever
possible. All of our book papers are acid-free, and our jackets and
covers are printed on paper with recycled content.

To the memory of Ged Bentley

Contents

Preface   ix

1 Washington and Its Academic Medical Centers   1
2 George Washington University: Selling the Hospital   5
3 George Washington University: Separating the Practice Plan   23
4 George Washington University: Closing the HMO   44
5 George Washington University and Its Medical School   49
6 Georgetown University: Selling the Hospital   80
7 Georgetown University: Selling the Practice Plan   108
8 Georgetown University and Its Medical School   128
9 MedStar Health   146
10 Conclusions   171

Appendix A: Other Universities with Teaching Hospitals Owned
    by For-Profit Companies   183
Appendix B. Reducing Deficits and Increasing Surpluses in
    Private Medical Schools That Do Not Own Their Primary
    Teaching Hospitals   192
Appendix C. Interviewees   204
Notes   233
Index   255

Photographs follow pages 79, 145, and 170.

Preface

When academic medical centers lose money, "attention must be paid." Two such institutions that found themselves floundering in red ink in the 1990s were the medical enterprises at George Washington (GW) and Georgetown universities, both in Washington, D.C. At their worst, GW lost $52 million in a three-year period during the decade, and Georgetown lost $83.1 million in 1999 alone.

Unable to repair the losses by themselves, both decided to sell their teaching hospitals—the biggest source of their troubles—and separate from the practice plans for their full-time faculties. Was this wise? What have been the effects of these decisions?

To answer these and other questions, I interviewed 335 people (see appendix C), some more than once, on the telephone, in their offices, or via e-mails, as I have done for my previous studies of academic medical centers.[1-3] I recorded what they told me by taking notes, not with a recorder. I sent all those interviewed drafts of what I wrote about them for correction and revision. This technique reduced the number of mistakes this book might otherwise contain and gave my interviewees the security of knowing that they would not see in print information they gave me in confidence. In some cases, they let me retain what they said but requested not to be identified as the source.

My journalist daughter, Elizabeth Kastor, has taken me to task for using this technique. The first time that most people interviewed for newspapers or magazines see what they have said is when they read about it. That would not work for my reports. Many of the sources would have remained silent if they had been unable to review the text that included their remarks. With this technique, almost everyone I contacted talked with me. Perhaps knowing that their interviewer was a fellow medical academic also put them at ease.

The book consists of ten chapters and three appendixes. In chapter 1, I describe how being located in Washington, D.C., affects the George Washington and Georgetown medical schools and their hospitals. Four chapters about George Washington and three chapters about Georgetown follow. Chapter 9 describes MedStar Health, the company that bought the Georgetown University Hospital and the medical school's faculty practice plan. In the final chapter, I review the lessons that I believe can be learned from the study. Appendix A covers the past and current statuses of those universities, other than George Washington, whose teaching hospitals are owned by for-profit companies. In appendix B, I review what I have learned about how a dean can reduce a structural deficit in a school of medicine. The names and titles of those interviewed are listed in appendix C.

I thank all those who allowed me to interview them. Without their help, this study could not have been conducted. I am particularly indebted to the interviewees who reviewed and commented on parts or all of the chapters. I thank the senior officers at the institutions studied who encouraged me in this project: at George Washington—Stephen Trachtenberg, president, and Dr. John Williams, vice president for health affairs; at Georgetown—John DeGioia, president, and Dr. Stuart Bondurant, interim executive vice president for health sciences and executive dean; and at MedStar Health—John McDaniel, CEO. Laura Cavender and Karen Alcorn at Georgetown and John Marzano at MedStar were particularly helpful.

I am very pleased that the Johns Hopkins University Press is publishing this volume, as it has two of my previous books. At the Press, I thank Wendy Harris, the medical editor, Maria denBoer, who edited the manuscript, and Becky Hornyak, who prepared the index. Phyllis Farrell, at the University of Maryland, the mistake-finder for all my books, read the proof and corrected the errors. Any that remain are my responsibility.

Selling Teaching Hospitals and Practice Plans

CHAPTER ONE

Washington and Its Academic Medical Centers

Washington, D.C., has long had three academic medical centers associated with three local universities—George Washington (GW),* Georgetown, and Howard. Until the past decade, each medical school owned its teaching hospital.† Although none of these medical schools is a leading research institution, each provides important clinical care for the district's citizens and trains medical students and graduate physicians that the region and the nation need. In 1997, GW agreed to sell its hospital to a for-profit hospital-owning corporation in Pennsylvania, and three years later Georgetown sold its teaching hospital to a Maryland-based not-for-profit corporation.‡ Both also separated from their practice plans for full-time clinicians.

Georgetown's and GW's schools of medicine have long faced problems that many other schools have not.[1-3] Although the federal government supports Howard for its role in training African American health care workers,

*Because everyone at George Washington University seems to use the acronym GW, I will do so also.

†Howard still owns its hospital.

‡For-profit companies are also called "investor-owned" companies.

the district government provides no financial help to either Georgetown's or GW's academic medical center.[4] In most states, the state-owned medical schools and teaching hospitals receive sizeable subventions. Many state legislatures also allocate funds to private universities for particular medical projects of importance to their respective states.

Compounding their financial woes, neither GW's nor Georgetown's medical center has developed an endowment comparable to those of other private academic medical centers. The problems became so severe that some feared that either or both of the medical schools might have to close.[5]

The Environment

Washington is a city in which the difference in wealth among its population of 575,000 is particularly striking. More than 70 percent of Washington residents are African American. Many are desperately poor, depending on Medicaid—if they qualify—to pay for their medical care. In the jargon of health care economics, Washington has a poor "payer mix." Compounding the demographics, "its government provides less support for the care of indigent patients than do many state governments," says Phillip Schaengold, a former executive at the George Washington University Hospital.[6]

At the other end of the economic spectrum are older, childless, wealthy citizens who can go to any medical center they choose, and Baltimore's famous Johns Hopkins Hospital is less than an hour away when the traffic is calm.[4,5]* The military hospitals, Walter Reed Army Medical Center and the National Naval Medical Center in Bethesda, Maryland, drain service personnel and elected federal officials from the private centers.[7] The city has its share of young, healthy professional and business couples who are gentrifying older sections of the city but need relatively little hospital care.[5]

"As for patients from Virginia," says Thomas Chapman, former George Washington University Hospital CEO, "we're separated by the 'Potomac Ocean.' Virginia people just don't come into DC for their health care."[5] As one of the George Washington clinical chairmen put it, "DC's an island be-

---

*"If we were in Montana, we might make it," comments a longtime executive of Washington medical institutions.

tween two states [Maryland and Virginia]."[8] Many potential patients from the suburbs are uneasy about driving into a city with a reputation for more than its share of crime.[4]

Even though the population of the city has decreased as former residents move to the suburbs, Washington retains its three medical schools.[4] "The district has more schools per resident than many other places," Chapman observes. "We're a city of two hundred-bed hospitals except for the Washington Hospital Center. I wondered where the patients would come from and how they would pay when the mayor was supporting building a new hospital for Howard to run. DC's not a healthy environment for health care financing."[5] Medicine is simply not Washington's predominant priority. "DC is a political city," says a former CEO of the George Washington University Hospital. "What's there is there. As for a stable health care market? Ha!"[6]

Once Washington achieved local governance in the 1970s, federal support for GW's and Georgetown's academic medical centers ceased,[4] as the district's budgets were continually stretched. Its support of Medicaid was severely reduced.[9,10] The hospitals also had to cope with the dropping payments for care by the insurers, culminating in the Balanced Budget Act of 1997, with its severe reductions in reimbursement by Medicare. Hospitals in the district lacked the advantages of the system of regulated hospital rates in nearby Maryland. The days when hospitals were "cash cows"—under the "cost-plus" system of compensation much admired by hospital executives and medical school leaders—were over.[10,11]

"Although an affluent city," comments Warren Greenberg, professor of health policy at GW, "Washington doesn't have many big corporations with people making large incomes" who can contribute significant amounts to institutions like the district's medical centers.[9] Many of Washington's most influential citizens are transient, which reduces their commitment to local institutions.[10]

Nevertheless, the city and surrounding communities, where many members of the medical faculties live, have many attractions—excellent schools in the suburbs and, in the city, free museums, music, theater, and a variety of restaurants whose quality is constantly improving. The National Institutes of Health (NIH) in nearby Bethesda, Maryland, provides a pool of nationally recognized medical investigators with whom scientists in the medical schools can collaborate and from which faculty can be recruited without requiring them to leave their homes. One longtime GW faculty member calls the region "the center of the scientific world."[12]

Medical Practice in Washington

No single hospital system or physician group dominates medical care in Washington, where strong community hospitals in the city and suburbs compete with the academic medical centers. Most doctors are in private practice and admit their patients to local hospitals. George Washington currently depends on and Georgetown in the past depended on privately practicing physicians to fill many of the beds in their university hospitals.

"Despite having many sophisticated, intelligent, well-paid residents, there seems to be a surprising lack of emphasis on being admitted to an academic medical center when you're sick," observes Dr. John LaRosa.[4] Drawing on his twenty-four years as a member of the GW medical faculty and from several years as one of its deans, LaRosa compares this attitude with that in New York and Boston, where the reputation of the medical school hospitals is high. Moreover, LaRosa comments, of those in the wealthier northern suburbs who do favor academic medical centers for their care, Johns Hopkins is not that much farther from where they live than are the medical centers in downtown Washington.[4]*

So, let us look at the medical centers at Georgetown and George Washington and study why they had to sell their teaching hospitals and practice plans, and what have been the effects of these decisions.

*LaRosa is president of the State University of New York Downstate Medical Center in Brooklyn and previously was chancellor of the Tulane University Medical Center in New Orleans.

CHAPTER TWO

George Washington University

Selling the Hospital

In the mid-1990s, The George Washington University* resolved to begin divesting itself of its hospital,† full-time physicians' practice plan, and health maintenance organization (HMO). Each was losing money—the medical center, as a whole, $52 million during a particularly difficult three-year period in the early 1990s.[3] The trustees and administration, after reviewing the problem in a retreat in the spring of 1995, decided to separate the university from the clinical enterprise and give the surviving entities "a way to navigate apart from what the university does."[3] The GW leaders realized they could not do everything at once, so they staged the process by selling the hospital in 1997, then separating from the practice plan in 2000, and finally closing the HMO two years later. They had decided that "throwing incremental dollars at the medical center wouldn't help."[3]

GW kept its medical school although, as president Stephen Joel Trachten-

---

*The federal charter established the name of the university as *The* George Washington University.[1] For convenience, I will drop the "The" in referring to the university.

†See the study by David Blumenthal and Joel Weissman on the sale of three teaching hospitals to investor-owned corporations. One of the three is George Washington University Hospital.[2]

berg wrote, "If GW did not have a medical center we would not create one. It is too difficult. It is too risky. It is too unpredictable. It would be easier for the university to survive—and in fact thrive—without it."[4] These considerations, compounded by years of red ink, had left the medical faculty, as a senior official observed, "morally depressed."[5]

What to Do with the Old Hospital

The process of divestment began with the George Washington University Hospital, the institution that presented the greatest financial risk to the university.[3,6]

By the 1990s, GW's hospital, which had opened in 1948 and had long been undercapitalized,[3,7,8] had become outdated and inefficiently expensive to operate. When patients needed hospitalization, all too many of the clinical faculty's well-insured and wealthy patients asked not to be admitted to the antiquated facility.[9] Consequently, many of the voluntary faculty with privileges elsewhere sent their private patients to other hospitals. Meanwhile, the GW hospital continued to treat aging patients from its HMO and poorly insured younger patients from Washington and the suburbs.[10] The hospital and faculty had long provided care for all patients who came to them, regardless of financial resources.[11]

When Dr. Mark Rogers, then the chairman of anesthesiology at Johns Hopkins, visited GW in 1993, he found the emergency department, named for former president Ronald Reagan, who had been treated there when he was shot in 1981, "even worse than the old one we used to have at Hopkins."[12]

"They were doing trauma in a shoebox" is the way Daniel McLean, who became the hospital CEO in 2000, describes GW's department.[13] The staff there were caring for sixty thousand patients per year in a unit designed for half as many.[14] "It seemed that we were treating more patients per square feet of space than at any hospital I knew about," said Dr. Mark Smith, the chairman of emergency medicine at GW from 1984 to 1995.[15]

During Rogers's visit, the daily average census in the hospital was about 250 to 280 patients.[16] "It was clearly a small hospital for an academic medical center," he thought.[12] By the time McLean started as CEO, the census had fallen to about 180.[16]

It was a "tired old building," Dr. John Williams Jr., an anesthesiologist and intensivist and since 1997 the head of the medical center, remembers.[14]* There were few private rooms, and the two-bed and four-bed rooms were cramped.[17] The hospital was wired for the 1940s, so its air conditioning and sprinkler systems were obsolete,[18] and it was laden with asbestos.[19] On the obstetrics unit, "the area for laboring patients was very small and did not permit easy visiting by more than one person at a time," remembers John Larsen, the department chairman.[20] The operating rooms were too small and underutilized, and parking was difficult.[21]

To make the badly needed changes in the hospital would require the university to heavily invest in its medical center, which, since being created in 1971–72, had become the biggest component of the university,[11] with one-third of its resources and 50 percent of its operating expenses.[22]

In 1992, the university had tried to convince the federal government to fund half of the cost of the much-needed renovations. The university argued that, despite receiving no money from the city or federal government, the GW hospital was annually providing $30 million of free care to city residents.[23] Even with the assistance of an influential senator, GW's attempt to secure $50 million from the federal government failed.[24] Citing frustration that the city and federal governments had refused to support the hospital, several senior executives at the medical center resigned.[25]

The hospital was no longer the cash cow that it had been in 1989, when the medical center had a cash balance of about $50 million.[11] Most of this surplus had been produced by the then-profitable hospital and could be invested in medical center and university projects. "All the money did not go into Victorian literature," says John Zeglis, a trustee from 1989 to 2000. "Some of the favored projects were at the medical center."[26]

The diagnosis-related group (DRG) system had led to lower payments for many hospital-based procedures and treatments.[27] Medicare was paying less, and the district had stopped reimbursing hospitals for the care of indigent patients. When Washington closed the District of Columbia General Hospital, its municipal hospital, in 2001,[28] more poorly insured patients started coming to the clinics and emergency departments and for admission to the beds[7,13,14,29] of, in particular, Washington Hospital Center, Prince George's Hospital Center in Cheverly, Maryland, and GW.[29]

Whether or not the hospital was losing money by the mid-1990s de-

---

*Williams is universally known as "Skip," a nickname he acquired in his youth.

pends on whom one asks. The president,[30] the university's chief financial officer,[22] and the trustees[31] claim that it was. Dr. Keith Ghezzi, the hospital medical director and chief operating officer from 1994 to 1996, remembers that the hospital was in the red by only $4 to $5 million when he became interim medical director in 1993.[21] Thomas Chapman, the hospital CEO from 1994 to 1996, says "the hospital was breaking even despite the university and medical school scraping off their piece and the discounts we had to give to the HMO and the full-time doctors. And the university knew this."[32] Hospital leaders estimated this payment to equal $40 to $50 million per year.[33] As one of the faculty, annoyed by the size of this and other similar transfers to the medical school and university, said, "If you questioned the amount, they'd say, 'It's just your share.' "*

Were the transfers a significant part of the problem? Opinions differ. The consensus among many physicians and administrators there at the time was that inappropriately large amounts of money were being transferred from the hospital to support the full-time physicians' practice plan and the HMO, both of which were in the red. Phillip Schaengold, the hospital CEO when the new owner took over in 1997, does not agree. "The transfers were not the problem. They were less than at some teaching hospitals I know about," he says. "Costs were too high, income was falling. They weren't investing in the hospital when it needed it.[7] Those were the real causes for the deteriorating situation, and they were the result of a less than effective senior management team."[35]

Whatever the size of the transfers, they were acceptable when the hospital was generating a surplus but as hospital income fell and expenses were inadequately controlled, the $50 million cash balance quickly disappeared.[8] Despite these events, the medical center continued to assign hospital funds to support losses at the practice plan and the HMO, though there is little agreement on how large they were. The practice plan needed the subsidy because many of its doctors were not earning enough to cover their expenses, some were being paid too generously, and the administra-

---

*That universities extract money from their medical centers will be familiar to all executives in such organizations, who usually hold that universities tax medical centers more than is appropriate. These are not, however, the only schools that universities consider profit centers. "The university milked the law school, which is a money maker," according to Sheldon Cohen, the distinguished tax lawyer who was commissioner of the Internal Revenue Service in the Johnson administration and taught in the GW law school for many years.[34] Cohen had received his undergraduate and law degrees from GW and was a trustee from 1980 and chairman when he retired from the board in 2001. As for "milking" funds from the law school, Trachtenberg denies that this occurred during his presidency.[1]

tion of the plan was inefficient. The effect of the transfers made the hospital's financial status seem worse than it would otherwise have appeared.

Having to use the university's personnel and administrative policies, many of which were not suited to the operations of a hospital, added to the cost of operating the hospital.[21] The university administration and some of the trustees questioned whether the hospital's leadership knew how to best manage its finances and operations.[22,34,36]

To develop the money for the renovations or replacement, the hospital would need to plead its case with the committee of the university trustees that governed the hospital and eventually with the whole board and the president. The project looked very expensive; it had to include a parking garage below the hospital. Despite the cost, however, the committee endorsed the replacement plan.[37]

After extensive discussion, the trustees[31] and the president, Stephen Trachtenberg,[30] rejected the proposal.[22] Trachtenberg believed that the replacement hospital would require too much capital and that the university should not take on the debt that financing a new hospital would require.* Furthermore, the project would compete with his plans for improving other schools and departments in the university. Though well known for the care it gave to President Reagan,† the hospital was "cash poor" as one of the hospital executives described its financial status.[37] "The capital just wasn't there," former hospital CEO Michael Barch remembers.[33]‡

---

*Dr. Floyd ("Fred") Loop, a GW medical graduate (class of 1962) and at the time CEO of the Cleveland Clinic Foundation, visited his old medical school in the early 1990s. "The hospital had very little debt. They could easily have financed the building of a 250-bed hospital," he remembers thinking.[38]

Delos ("Toby") Cosgrove, Loop's successor as chairman of thoracic and cardiovascular then and more recently as CEO of the Cleveland Clinic, also visited George Washington just before it was sold. The Clinic and GW discussed forming a clinical collaboration in the specialty. Cosgrove concluded, however, that in meeting with GW officers, he was "talking with the wrong people" in view of the imminent sale and terminated the negotiations.[39]

†Dennis O'Leary, the doctor who held the news conferences at the time and became the public's contact with the hospital, called Reagan's hospitalization "a real tonic for the staff. It really put us on the map, gave us much recognition, so that people no longer thought us second to Georgetown in academic medicine in Washington." Commenting on the extent of Reagan's injuries, O'Leary says, "The actor and the actress needed to believe that he almost died, but he didn't. It also served the interest of the White House to portray Reagan as a hero who had miraculously escaped death."[40]

In commemoration of the president's hospitalization, the emergency department was named the Reagan Institute. The university, however, has not realized as much as it might have from the connection. Though GW raised most of the money, some of Reagan's associates helped, "but most of them are either gone or have developed other interests," says Dr. Robert Shesser, the chairman of the department. "Looking forward, we may eventually change its name to the 'Presidential Institute.'"[41]

‡Barch is now chairman of the board of Global Pharmaceutical Sourcing, Bethesda, Maryland.

"Although a deliberate strategy," Louis Katz, executive vice president and treasurer of the university, observed, selling the hospital "was not a popular decision."[22] There were some members of the board,[42] remembers Robert Perry, a longtime trustee and for many years chairman of the committee assigned to the medical center, "who were quite emotional about selling. It was as if George Washington had been born there."[36]

Despite objections and sentiment, the only solution, Trachtenberg concluded, was to sell the hospital to a buyer that would do what he felt the university could not afford to do. One of the executives remembered Trachtenberg saying, "All I see is risks associated with the hospital."[33] Trachtenberg wanted the university out of the clinical business, which he saw as a current and future drain on the university's finances, and limit the university's involvement in medicine to education and research, activities that he thought less risky than the other elements of GW's medical enterprise. He told a colleague, "University presidents shouldn't be in the hospital business. Their skills lie elsewhere."[43]

Trachtenberg worried that the medical school and its hospital, full-time faculty's practice plan, and HMO would become increasingly onerous burdens for the university,[14,36,44] eventually draining the income and even the corpus of the endowment.[45] As trustee chairman Charles Manatt put it, "There was a clear and present danger that the losses would eat the endowment."[45]* As for the university hospital, Trachtenberg had concluded, "We don't know much about running a hospital, and we're not very good at it."[31] He reminded the trustees, "It's not our core business."[46] The trustees unanimously supported Trachtenberg's advice to sell the hospital.[31] Trustee Robert Perry praised the president. "Steve had the fortitude to make the hard decisions."[36]

Selling the Hospital

Selling the GW hospital in the mid-1990s was not a new idea. Ten years previously, the possibility had been considered[47] because of fears about how the advent of managed care would affect its financial welfare. "There were serious discussions," remembers Patricia Gurne, the vice chairman of

---

*Vice chairman of the trustees Patricia Gurne remembers that "the operative word about the hospital at this time was 'hemorrhaging.' "[46]

the board, "but we didn't trust the buyer, and so the board rejected the offer."[46] The company also withdrew after concluding that George Washington's asking price was too high.[47]

By 1995, GW believed that the property it wanted to sell would now appear attractive to potential buyers. "Our clinician faculty, which was very good, and the hospital served most of the VIPs in Washington," Barch remembered.[33] "We had all the component pieces on the clinical side."[33]

The university proceeded to solicit potential buyers. Several proposals came from for-profit hospital-owning companies, none of which was accepted.* The hospital rejected one company because "we felt that we could not keep appropriate control of the academics."[33] Furthermore, selling to one of the for-profit companies required that the District of Columbia issue a certificate of need (CON), which specifically discouraged such purchases.[48] Critics of GW's sale to a for-profit company warned that if such a company bought the hospital without a CON, "vital but expensive services may be eliminated without public view," as *Modern Healthcare* magazine reported.[48]

Medlantic, the Washington- and Maryland-based not-for-profit hospital-owning company,† which was bidding for the George Washington University Hospital,[49] bought advertisements objecting to any change in the CON law that would benefit the for-profits.[48] Medlantic favored legislation that would open the details of all such deals to public scrutiny and ensure that charitable assets were properly valued.[50] One of the district's council members proposed that $5 million—a number that the sponsor admitted was an arbitrary figure—be imposed on all sales of not-for-profit hospitals to for-profit companies. The final version of the bill required that any hospital sold in the district would pay the city 10 percent of its real estate taxes for the previous five years, which came, at the time, to about $500,000 for GW.[51]

GW executives responded that "Medlantic [was] being 'protectionist' and that the regulations involved with obtaining a CON [were] keeping healthcare resources out of Washington."[48] Medlantic's intense lobbying campaign, which *The Washington Post* called "unprecedented for a city medical institution," tried to persuade the public and the district's govern-

---

*The university had considered selling the hospital to a for-profit company as early as the 1970s.[17]

†Medlantic, later renamed MedStar Health, would eventually buy the Georgetown University hospital. (See chapter 6.)

ment that a for-profit hospital would refuse to provide its fair share of medical care for the poor.[51]

Very troubling to many at GW was the rumor that Medlantic, if it became the successful buyer, would close the University Hospital and move the inpatient facilities to the campus of the Washington Hospital Center,[51,52] Medlantic's flagship institution in north Washington, several miles from the main GW campus. Downtown, only the medical office buildings, outpatient surgery, and an emergency room would be retained.[49] The chief of cardiology at GW remembered thinking, "We would be turned into emergency docs who transferred all our sick patients to the Washington Hospital Center."[53]*

Full-time members of the GW clinical faculty looked on the Washington Hospital Center as a solely clinical operation, and believed that, in the words of a GW loyalist, "no one in the academic community trusted it."[53] And then there were the politics of who would hold the senior jobs of division chiefs and department chairmen if GW merged with the owners of the hospital center.[53]

GW doctors were not alone in criticizing a possible union with Medlantic. The district's council chairman said, "Medlantic just wanted the hospital to be closed, but we had to look at what was best for the citizens of the District of Columbia."[51]

One person at GW who felt less uncomfortable about Medlantic buying the hospital, however, was the university president Stephen Trachtenberg. He visualized building new medical school buildings on the Washington Hospital Center campus, where space was available, and transferring the entire GW medical enterprise there. "Nobody but me liked the idea," Trachtenberg said.[1] Nothing came of it.

By October 1996, the news about town was that GW would sell the hospital to the Nashville-based for-profit company, OrNda HealthCorp, the nation's third largest hospital-owning company with fifty hospitals, mostly in the Southwest. George Washington University Hospital would be its first academic medical center.[54] However, OrNda was then in the process of merging with Tenet Healthcare, the second largest for-profit hospital company.[54] Although the proposal interested the GW leaders, they became un-

---

*This is what happened to cardiology at the Georgetown University Hospital after MedStar bought it. (See chapter 6.)

comfortable about selling while the structure of the company was changing.[37] As for Tenet, it preferred buying the St. Louis University Hospital, which, unlike GW's hospital, was profitable, and was questioning the wisdom of purchasing two university hospitals at the same time.[52]

When Tenet decided not to buy the George Washington University Hospital, GW imposed a forty-five-day "veil of secrecy." During this hiatus, morale fell,[19] and, according to Dr. Allan Weingold, the vice president for medical affairs at the time, "the faculty hovered on suicide. With hat-in-hand, we went back to Universal [Universal Health Services, Inc. of King of Prussia, Pennsylvania] who had submitted a bid to buy the hospital."[10] In April 1997, Universal bought an 80 percent interest in the hospital, with GW retaining 20 percent.* District Partners, LLP, was created as a limited partnership that would own the hospital on behalf of the two principals.[22]

Universal, seen by the GW officials as a stable company,[37] was, like Tenet, a for-profit hospital-owning corporation.† The deal prescribed that Universal share power with GW on the governing board of District Partners, LLC,[22,56] with GW retaining ownership of the land.[22] The board of directors of the joint venture would assume authority over the hospital's medical services. Each partner would have equal representation, thereby assuring, theoretically at least, that the hospital would maintain its academic mission and continue to serve indigent patients.[57,58] All decisions would require agreement by a majority of the trustees, giving the university a veto on issues it considered vital to the hospital's mission. The hospital's twelve-member board of trustees would remain in place and supervise accreditation, quality assurance, and service delivery. At least seven of its members would come from the community.[57] Universal agreed to assume management of the hospital immediately.

Universal paid $125 million for its purchase, with most of the money allocated to capital improvements at the hospital. About $80 million would be spent "at once" and $45 million during the next ten years.[57]‡ Universal also pledged to offer jobs to all hospital employees and retain existing services.[56] Particularly attractive to the medical center and university officials was Universal's agreeing that if the hospital lost money, the corporation,

---

*MedStar had not offered GW the 80:20 deal that Universal proposed.[52]

†About 15 percent of U.S. hospitals are for-profit.[55]

‡Critics quickly complained that the $125 million was inadequate to successfully renovate the hospital.[59] At this point, a replacement hospital was not on the table.

not the university, would pay. If the hospital made a profit, the university would get 20 percent of it, in keeping with its share of the ownership.[14] Attractive as these terms appeared, some of the trustees worried that, if the finances turned bleak, Universal might call for capital from the university. Also, would the company skimp on providing services and equipment requested by the faculty?[26]*

Tom Chapman, the last hospital director before Universal bought it, said, "Despite the university's pessimistic analysis of the hospital's financial past and concerns about its future, Universal saw it having economic value, and, of course, prestige." Chapman knew Universal was a financially successful company and a careful purchaser. "They insist on seeing some 'green.' Nevertheless, I do not think Universal fully understood how tough it would be to succeed in this large, difficult market."[32]

Medlantic, the local not-for-profit company, was not happy. "GW has engaged in bait-and-switch tactics that play Russian roulette with the community's health," one of its officers complained.[56] The fee that the district assigned to purchasers, however, pleased Medlantic. "A very significant step in recognizing the need for regulatory oversight of these transactions," said one of its executives.[51]

The hospital and Universal, however, were exempted from the provisions of the new legislation that required for-profit buyers and not-for-profit sellers to disclose the details of transactions to the district's corporation counsel for review.[60] They would, however, be required to pay about $600,000 in back property taxes and continue to spend the same amount of money on uncompensated care to the poor—$19.9 million in 1996—for the next five years.[60] In retrospect, Weingold says, "We made a mistake not taking Universal originally."[10]

Why Did Universal Buy the Hospital?

The CEO of Universal Health Services is Alan Miller, who founded the company in 1978. Miller had previously worked in advertising and been chairman and president of American Medicorp until that company was sold to a larger hospital-owning corporation. By 2005, the corporation that Mil-

---

*Some of the physicians would later argue that this concern was valid. (See below.)

ler now led owned ninety-one facilities, of which twenty-four are acute care hospitals and the others behavioral health, ambulatory surgery, and radiation oncology treatment centers. Its annual revenue is about $4 billion.[55]

Universal, however, had had no experience with academic medical centers or hospitals in large cities like Washington.[56,59] Most of its acute care hospitals are located in cities and towns in California, Florida, Texas, and Nevada, where the population is growing and hospitals are needed. It is Universal's policy to acquire hospitals only where there are no more than one or two competitors so that the company can dominate their markets with as much as 30 to 40 percent of the business. In the Northeastern and Midwestern states, where the population is either stable or decreasing, Universal has few acute care hospitals. "These places have all the hospitals they need, "Miller explained.*

Although in buying the GW hospital, Universal would acquire one of the largest hospitals the company then owned, it was a hospital in a community where the population was dropping, where there were many competing hospitals, and where the hospital then served no more than 15 percent of the market.[22] In addition to acquiring its first university hospital,† Universal would be the first out-of-town firm to buy a major hospital in the district.[59]

So why did Universal buy the hospital? Despite its problems, George Washington University Hospital had several advantages for any potential buyer: it was the only hospital in its immediate location, the real estate was favorable, and its business was predictable.

"We wanted to be in the nation's capital," Miller explains. The location would bring the company closer to Congress and to the lobbying efforts of the for-profit hospital trade association. Suitable accommodations for VIP patients and their security guards were available. The treatments that Ronald Reagan and Dick Cheney received at George Washington have been widely publicized, and President George W. Bush has used visits to the hospital to announce health care initiatives. "When for-profits are mentioned, we get good press," Miller said.[55]

The prestige of owning its first university hospital was another attrac-

*I interviewed Miller three weeks after Hurricane Katrina had flooded the two acute care hospitals Universal owns in Louisiana.
†Allan Weingold from GW quipped, "Shows how much they knew."[10]

tion, to "enhance its image," said Phillip Schaengold, CEO and managing director of the hospital from 1997 to 2000.[61] The company hoped to use the hospital's educational mission to train doctors and administrators from its other hospitals with methods that would help the company's community hospitals prosper.

But owning the George Washington University Hospital would not be the same for Universal as owning community hospitals. "Though we saw it as an opportunity, it's been difficult," Miller admits. "Employing doctors is not like employing others. Academics and running a business are not necessarily an easy fit. The hospital is very resource consuming, and we must accept a lower return than for our other hospitals." All of which has convinced Miller that Universal should not buy another teaching hospital.[55]

A New Hospital

When Universal assumed its 80 percent ownership of the George Washington University Hospital, it appointed Phillip Schaengold to be CEO and managing director in April 1997. Schaengold came to Washington from Detroit, where he had been president and CEO of the Sinai Health System. He found an old hospital with more than its share of problems and worked to improve financial management, purchasing, marketing, and billing and collections. "The infrastructure—information technology particularly—was behind the times," he found. "The hospital was suffering from benign neglect."[7]

Using Universal's capital, the new team "cleaned up the old hospital and spruced it up." Universal added new technology—scanners for radiology, a new cardiac catheterization laboratory—which could be transferred into a new hospital, if building one was the eventual decision. The new management also renovated the outmoded obstetrics floor.

In February 1998, less than a year after declaring that the George Washington University Hospital would be renovated, not replaced, the university and Universal announced that they would build a new four hundred-bed hospital in a university-owned parking lot across Twenty-third Street from the old hospital,[62] a solution that many at GW saw as inevitable.[18] This was not well received by Medlantic and its Washington Hospital Center, "which opposed granting a certificate of need (CON) that we needed to replace rather than convert the old hospital," Schaengold remembers.[7]* The same institutions had opposed the CON that GW required to convert the hospital from not-for-profit to for-profit status.[7]

This fortuitously located site meant that patients could continue to be cared for in the old hospital until the new building was ready to receive them. If renovation had been the decision, the construction would have had to be carried out in the same building where patients were being treated. Though licensed for 501 beds, the old hospital was operating only about 250 beds, not all of which were usually filled with patients.[13]

Several limitations prevented building a hospital with as many beds as the old hospital had, even if that had been desirable:[13,36]

- The size of the new lot was smaller than the old one, and, despite building out to the street lines, each floor would have less space.
- Height was limited by proximity to the White House.
- Building a garage below the building was prevented by the presence of the Metro subway there.
- Private rooms were now essential rather than the more space-efficient, multi-bed units in the old hospital.

And there were problems particular to the neighborhood. Conflict was endemic between the university and the residents of the area,[7] some of whom had vociferously objected to the noise created by the large diesel trucks bringing supplies to the old hospital while they were waiting on the streets to enter the loading dock. "I remember them monitoring, minute by minute, how long the trucks were there," says Dan McLean when he became CEO of the old hospital in 2000.[13] These complaints forced the hospital to unload its supplies at another location and then transport the cargoes in smaller vehicles to the hospital, an inefficient and expensive solution that was abandoned in the new hospital.[13] The community then sued to prevent the use of loading docks at the new hospital. Although the court threw out the suit, legal fees cost the company about $500,000.[13]

The cost to build the new six-story hospital was estimated at $96 million, between $800 and $900 per square foot,[10] significantly less than $150 million, the upwardly revised figure that renovating the old hospital might

*Schaengold is now executive director of the University Hospital at the State University of New York (SUNY) Upstate Medical University in Syracuse.

cost. Each room would be private, a marked change from the existing hospital in which 80 percent of the rooms accommodated more than one patient. In an effort to compete successfully with community hospitals, the obstetrics floor would include facilities so that the newborns' fathers could stay overnight.[62]

As expected, the competition complained that, with nearly one in three hospital beds in Washington vacant during most of 1997,[63] the new hospital would only add to the problem. As *The Washington Post* reported: "The plan illustrates what health economists call a 'medical arms race.' In communities that have more hospital capacity than they need, hospitals fighting for survival often respond by investing in even more plant and equipment."[62]

Many local health care executives had nominated George Washington University Hospital as the one that would close. With a new modern hospital coming, "somebody's going to have to come up with another nominee as to who's going down," observed a New York investment banker who had advised the university.[62] The construction went forward, and the new hospital opened in July 2002. Transferring the patients across Twenty-third street into the new building took only twelve hours.

By 2006, the new George Washington University Hospital's daily census ran about 250 patients.* The hospital is staffed for 260 beds and registered for 325, fewer than in the original plans and less than university officials had originally wanted.[3] Should demand require, the administration can "flex the staff" to accommodate 300 patients by bringing in extra nurses.[64]

The beds are organized around four-room pods, each with its own nurse and computer. There is an intensive care unit (ICU) on each of the three medical and surgical floors. Each takes patients from any specialty, not a universally popular practice among all the faculty, some of whom prefer specialized ICUs.[19]

Although most of the faculty did not favor selling the hospital—university officials believe they feared losing control if the hospital was no longer a part of George Washington University[22]—most of them now agree that the sale was wise,[10,14,17-19,44,65-72] as does the university's leadership.[3,73,74] To the amazement of some of the more academic faculty, Universal has proved

---

*The payer mix in 2006 was approximately 33 percent managed care (HMO/PPO [preferred provider organization]), 33 percent Medicare, 12 percent Medicaid and indigent, and the rest commercial.

to be a good partner.[29,53,65,66,75-77] Private patients like the new hospital—the deficiencies of the old place drove them away—and Universal runs it better than the university did.[18,19,65,74] "They've [Universal] behaved very nicely," according to Allan Weingold.[10] However, opinions differ about Universal and the academic mission. Weingold believes "they recognize the academic commitment";[10] others are not so sure.[70,78]

As for a for-profit company owning 80 percent of its university hospital, vice president John Williams believes GW is much better off. "There's greater discipline now among the doctors, trainees, and students when it comes to ordering unnecessary tests and procedures." Williams has found Universal "very responsive to our capital needs."[14]

Because the administration seemed wedded to the idea of ridding the university of its money-losing, renovation-needing hospital, better that an out-of-town company, using corporate money to repair or replace the hospital and willing to share its future with the university, become the purchaser. All agree that this was a wiser solution than merging with a local company like Medlantic, which might close the university hospital and move much of the clinical work to a hospital with less emphasis on academic work.

"All of a sudden there was investment of capital," one senior member of the faculty said. "It's nice to have a partner with deep pockets."[53] In 2004 alone, the hospital spent $12 million on capital improvements. Dr. Michael Seneff, who directs the intensive care units, agrees. "Before Universal, the answer was always 'no.' Now, though we have to put together persuasive reasons to buy this or that, the answer's usually 'yes.' "[19]

Universal is pleased with its decision to buy GW's hospital, which, in fiscal year 2005, had an 8 percent operating margin (surplus) on net revenue of $275 million. Since the new hospital opened, it has never lost money on operations,[14] and will soon construct a new building for outpatients. As part of a for-profit corporation that pays taxes, the George Washington University Hospital cannot accept gifts, so philanthropy from the patients must be solicited by the medical school.

A New Broom

Acquisition of the hospital by a private company brought to GW a chief executive who had never previously worked in an academic medical center, making him inexperienced according to his critics but unbiased according to him. The new CEO was Daniel McLean, an Air Force Academy graduate who earned an M.S. in health care administration (cum laude) at the University of Houston at Clear Lake and lists swimming, skiing, aerobics, golf, and travel as "special skills and interests" in his résumé.* He had worked his way up in hospital administration, and when transferred to GW, was CEO and managing director of Universal's McAllen Medical Center, a 490-bed tertiary hospital that serves the upper Rio Grande Valley from McAllen, Texas.

The customs of academic administration were, to put it mildly, different from what he was used to. "Historically, at the university, political power and authority are everything."[13] McLean was amazed at the degree to which finances between the medical school and hospital had been intertwined. "All the dollars went into one pot," he discovered. "Whoever got there first and had the biggest hands got the money. The hospital was paying the medical school $1 million annually for use of its library. Outrageous! We got it down to $250,000—still more than appropriate for this service."[13]

McLean thought that the best word to describe the administration of the medical center when he arrived was "anarchy."[13] McLean found that many of the chairmen of the clinical departments did not know what their jobs as service chiefs entailed and decided to evaluate the quality of their leadership at the hospital.† This was his practice at the community hospitals where, up until then, he had always worked. He criticized their "avoiding budgets and trying to hire people without following appropriate HR [human resources] protocols and declared that unilateral business decisions would not be tolerated."[13]

"How dare you?" the chiefs complained.‡ "So, with the assistance of the hospital's medical director, we drew up job descriptions for the chiefs of service and told them that management expected the chiefs to pay attention to such matters as standards of care and quality management on their

---

*For whatever it may say about McLean's experience with physicians, both of his sons became doctors. When he left GW in 2004, McLean returned to Texas as group director of Universal's seven hospitals and eight hundred beds in the South Texas Region and CEO of the South Texas Health System.

†As is traditional in many medical schools, the chairmen of the clinical departments also direct the relevant services at the university hospital.

‡"I'm surprised you didn't hear the roar at Maryland," McLean said referring to the medical school in Baltimore where I work.[13]

services." Some responded, "I don't know how to do these things," or "I haven't got the staff to do it." "So," McLean responded, "then how can you be expected to direct a hospital department?"[13]

McLean made it clear that the hospital had the right to approve the performance of each chief and could reject those who could not perform. "It was a shock to them to be told that they had obligations to the hospital and to the other chiefs. Silos were the rule. There was no cross-pollination."[13] When the chiefs would not or could not assume these duties, rather than try to push them out, the hospital engaged voluntary faculty on a part-time basis to help.[13] Using funds supplied by the hospital, the medical school pays them directly and not through the full-time clinical departments.[8]

Faculty versus Universal

Despite appreciating the obvious advantage of Universal's building a new plant to serve their patients, faculty members have faulted some of Universal's plans. On one occasion, the business interests of the company conflicted with the professional standards of the faculty. Universal wanted to establish a service in which children with conduct disorders would be housed in the new hospital. The company's rationale for the service was that there was a neurological basis for the disorders that could be studied by the faculty. Universal wanted the psychiatry department's chairman to staff it.

"The data supporting the concept were very soft," says Dr. David Reiss, the department's leading investigator. "They were after federal dollars available for this work.[79] I don't recall that they made a serious offer to the faculty for research. There were no faculty members engaged in any of these issues, as research topics, at the time."[80] The doctors, joined by Skip Williams,[5] "raised hell," in Reiss's words, and the program was moved to a different facility.[65,79]

Another conflict between the psychiatry department and the new hospital's management involved Universal's desire to outsource the psychiatry services to a distant hospital, "which would have been horrible for our academic training program," said Dr. David Mrazek, the chairman at the time. Universal did not do this, but in Mrazek's opinion, "they made good on their pledge [to maintain an academic psychiatry service in the hospital], but minimally."[70] The psychiatry service in the hospital is quite small.

The senior partner of a large general surgical group,* which he character-izes as having been "embedded" in the George Washington University Hospital for decades, finds several problems:

- *Staff attitudes,* about which his patients often complain. This is a longstanding problem and explains why some doctors do not want to admit there despite the new building. "You're interfering with my day" seems to be the general attitude rather than "what can I do to help. It's an attitude of mediocrity."
- *The building.* "The public spaces are great but, for example, the surgeons' lockers were too small" until the group forced a change. There are no on-call rooms for the house staff who sleep and hang out "in tiny spaces,"† and, he says, "there are not enough elevators." The physical design leaves no opportunity for growth if that should become desirable.
- *Operating rooms.* "As a starter, there are not enough of them." Long halls, a characteristic architectural feature throughout the hospital, are particularly inefficient on the operating room floor. Functionally, the surgeons complain about the long "turnover time" needed to clean and prepare the operating rooms, leaving the surgeons to find ways to fill their time while waiting to do their next case.
- *Consulting the doctors.* When Universal was planning the building, "they never asked us how to do it," and he is not the only doctor making this complaint.

---

*Who prefers to remain anonymous.

† When space became available as the census dropped, "the residents took over the old hospital," said Daniel McLean, the first CEO of the new hospital building. Now this luxury is no longer available. "The on-call rooms we built are small, but they're adequate. They have single accommodations, TVs, and computers," but, McLean admits, may not be adjacent to the areas where the residents' patients were located. The departments must share the use of the conference rooms.[13] There had been space in the old hospital for medical students to sleep. In the new building, these facilities are not provided nor are they required by the agreement between the school of medicine and the hospital owners.

CHAPTER THREE

George Washington University

Separating the Practice Plan

Medical Faculty Associates, Inc.

On July 1, 2000, George Washington University and the medical center spun off Medical Faculty Associates (MFA), its practice plan for the full-time clinical faculty, into a separate, not-for-profit, tax-exempt 501(c)(3) corporation.[1] GW wanted to remove itself as much as possible from responsibility for an operation that, in view of its previous financial problems, could jeopardize the fiscal well-being of the university and its medical school in the future.

When first proposed, the faculty seemed to favor "being their own bosses," remembers Louis Katz, the university executive vice president. "They wanted autonomy and more money."[2] Later, however, they had second thoughts.[3,4] "I was nervous about splitting off," says Alan Wasserman, chairman of the practice plan and of the department of medicine.[4] Many predicted that the new enterprise would fail. Some doctors felt that "MFA was being left out to dry."[5] The doctors realized, however, that if they opposed the separation, the medical school might try to decrease their compensation.[6]

The practice plan had been losing money, as much as $8 million in some years,[4] an amount that surprised and even "appalled"[7] the trustees. Some of the chairmen were paying their faculty and themselves bonuses even though their departments and the plan as a whole were in deficit. The number doing this, however, was not great, according to Skip Williams. "There were relatively few doctors being paid super-salaries before 2000," when MFA became independent.[8] The outdated university hospital added to MFA's financial woes by discouraging private patients from seeking care from the full-time physicians who admitted there.[2]

Management was undisciplined, with no one at the university, medical school, or practice plan exercising responsibility for departmental losses or for the overall financial status of the plan. As one of the trustees said, "The leadership at the medical school wouldn't lead* and the practice plan [when part of the university] couldn't repair itself."[10] No one would take responsibility for the unpleasant chore of disciplining or even relieving chairmen whose departments were insolvent, remembers Gerald Bass, the medical center's chief financial officer.[11]

"There were major back-office problems," Bass remembers.[11] The systems for billing and collecting that MFA was using were inefficient and antiquated.[12,13] Financial information needed to negotiate effectively for managed care contracts was unavailable. The university's human resources department, which MFA was obliged to use, restricted hiring the most competent staff and discharging underperforming workers.[14] Communications were inadequate. Patients phoning the MFA had to wait a long time to reach someone who could arrange appointments.[13]

As for the doctors, they were seen as lacking "get up and go," according to a trustee. "They were salaried without incentives to work harder and more efficiently."[15] A doctor who left GW for another job explained the financial problems this way: "Many of MFA's leaders were used to a subsidized system supported by the university, so they didn't work hard to bring in new business." So, thought another of the trustees, "let them fix it."[16]

When John Williams became the medical center's chief executive in 1997, he appointed Wasserman medical director of the practice plan, which was then a part of the medical school.[4] From 1997 to 1999, the first two years after the hospital was sold, the medical center, in Williams's words, "kept the doctors whole," but encouraged MFA to decrease salaries based

---

*MFA reported to the dean before it was separated from the school.[9]

on performance. "This didn't make Jerry* or me very popular," Williams remembers.[8]

Wasserman reports that the salaries were dropped by as much as 25 percent, even in departments that were solvent, which led to the departure of several doctors.[4] The equivalent of thirty full-time employees was reduced, mostly by attrition.[11] To cover the losses that remained after the cash had been spent, the medical center began borrowing from the university, which charged interest at 6.5 percent.[11]

Concluding that the practice plan was "its greatest risk," now that the hospital had been sold, the university decided to terminate its responsibility for this troublesome entity.[4] Only by giving the full-time doctors self-government, the school's leaders thought, would they assume effective responsibility for the plan's profits and losses.[11,17] Also, if the university could divest itself of the medical school's clinical practice, its executives thought —overly optimistically in retrospect—they would no longer have to listen to the complaints of the full-time clinical faculty about excessive "taxing" of practice earnings for overhead and other charges.[18,19]

Some of the university trustees threatened to close the medical school unless something was done about the losses in the practice plan, several faculty members and administrators told me.[4,11,20] Louis Katz denies that the university ever planned to do this or that he ever said that it would,[21] although faculty members insist that he did.†

Despite being dramatically stated, this was an empty threat. Trachtenberg had written: "Closing the medical school . . . [is] not an option. Having a medical enterprise is part of what makes us complete as an academic and intellectual organization. To sever it would diminish us in our own eyes and the eyes of the rest of the world."[23] Nevertheless, Trachtenberg was worried. "In the end what's missing," he e-mailed me after reviewing a draft of the manuscript, "was the terror of the moment—the feeling that the medical center, hospital, and medical school were going to fold. And it was going to happen on my watch. The contemplation of something like that focuses the mind and makes one uniquely alert."[23]

---

*Gerald Bass is the administrator whom Williams had recently appointed to repair the financial problems of the practice plan. Later, Bass moved into the vice president's office and became Williams's chief financial advisor.

†Katz arouses widely differing opinions in the medical school. Though many criticize him, he has his supporters like Skip Williams, who says, "He's very bright and really understands finance and economics. Lou's in effect the COO of university, and the trustees admire him."[22]

Structure

After prolonged negotiations and planning, a separate corporation, Medical Faculty Associates, Inc. was formed. The eleven-member, self-perpetuating[1] board of directors would consist, as it does today, of four department chairmen: one from medicine, one from surgery, one from the hospital-based departments, and one at large. Also on the board are the dean—the only representative of the medical school[1]—three faculty members who are not chairmen, and three outside members. Alan Wasserman, the medical director of the practice plan when it was part of the university, became president and chairman of the board of the newly independent MFA. When Gerald Bass became associate vice president for health economics in Williams's office, Stephen Badger was recruited as MFA's senior administrator with the title of CEO.[4] Badger reports to Wasserman, not to the dean.[24]

Wasserman is described as "a very fine negotiator and businessperson and on top of things"[10] and Badger as "bright and energetic, the best administrator by far that we have ever had. He has held our feet to the fire, which we badly needed."[27] Despite these skills and accomplishments, however, Badger has become the focus of significant antagonism from some of the current and former clinical chairmen who complain that he had become their boss rather than Wasserman or the dean. As one current chairman put it, "Despite Badger's unquestioned abilities, he is mostly a money manager who has little knowledge of the clinical operations. The budget seems to be all that matters. Alan [Wasserman] was very much involved in the day-to-day business of MFA early on but lately seems to have ceded this to Badger, who has enthusiastically taken it on. Badger seems to make many of the decisions now and, consequently, takes most of the heat."[25]*

The Doctors versus the University

Despite the separation, the clinicians continue to complain about issues, some of which will be familiar to all leaders in academic medicine:[4,6,24,26-31]

---

*Although I interviewed Stephen Badger, who provided very helpful information, he declined to review the relevant portions of the manuscript.

- *The dean's tax*—to which the plan's officers agreed without much enthusiasm—of 0.5 percent of gross collections starting the second year after the separation from the university and rising 0.5 percent per year until reaching a maximum of 3 percent.[1,11] Although this amount is smaller than what practice plans at many medical schools pay, it continues to rankle. The clinical department chairmen look in vain for the school to invest the tax in projects they favor.* As one of the chairmen complained, "Skip [John Williams, the executive vice president] and the dean disagree on the pledge the university made to us [about the dean's tax]. It's a very contentious issue. All our margin's going back to the university and medical school."

- *Payment for teaching by the school* that the clinical chairs believe inadequately compensates them for this duty.

- *Indirect payments* from federal grants developed by the doctors, none of which returns to the MFA.† They further complain that the university administers the grants poorly.

- *Outpatient imaging.* The hospital retains this facility, thereby depriving the departments of income from owning the equipment and billing for its use.

- *Firing underperforming chairmen.* "No one's willing or able to fire the chairs," one of the clinical chairmen complained. "They're just as unaccountable now as then."

- *Medical school–hospital relationships.* The doctors complain that the medical school will not help them "pressure" the hospital for "things that we want."

The Malpractice Trust

Upon separating from the medical center, MFA assumed funding the portion of the trust that supports claims against the doctors.‡ The medical center had carried this responsibility for both constituencies through a single malpractice trust before the hospital was sold and MFA was spun off.

---

*According to the university, the doctors have never presented a satisfactory business plan describing how they would use the funds.[2]

†MFA administers the pharmaceutical grants, but they pay less in indirect costs than federal grants do.

‡Universal deals with claims against the hospital.

The university insists that MFA build a large reserve, partly to pay for the "tail" since MFA became independent.* Although Washington, D.C., has "one of the worst malpractice situations in the country,"[31] the chairmen assert that the amount the university requires MFA to reserve is unrealistically high and reflects the university leaders' "risk-adverse obsession."† One of the chairmen described this requirement in Washingtonian terms as an "unfunded mandate." Consequently, the chairmen complain, "MFA will never make money."‡

The departments pay different amounts based on income rather than risk, a formula about which some of the chairmen complain. Allan Weingold adds, "MFA's malpractice costs are higher than for voluntary faculty, because we try to avoid jury trials, but it costs money to settle."[31] The school, members of the clinical faculty say, threatened to reduce MFA's support for education if the practice plan refused to increase the size of the malpractice reserve.

Independence or Dependence

Despite the hopes of the clinical leadership that a separate MFA would leave the doctors masters of their fate, the terms establishing MFA, members say:

- "We're dictated to by the university."
- "We lost on many major issues when MFA was set up."
- "We're a stepchild of the medical center."
- "It's a pyrrhic victory for the doctors since the details in the affiliation agreement so favor the university. We're held hostage to the university."

Theoretically, the medical school can control, or at least strongly influence, the actions that MFA takes if it chooses to do so.[1,6,27,31,33] The school

---

*The university funds the cost of suits that may arise over incidents occurring during the years when MFA was part of the medical center.[8]

†According to Louis Katz, three actuaries advised about how large the reserve should be. "Theirs [MFA's] said that it was overfunded. Ours [the university's] and the independent actuary said it was underfunded."[2] At the medical school, Williams and Bass insist that the reserve is appropriate.[8,12] Katz believes, despite the objections of the leaders of MFA, that malpractice suits pose a serious threat to the financial well-being of MFA and the university and that maintaining a large reserve is essential.[32]

‡If they had these funds, one of the chairmen told me, they would spend the money to hire a better-paid and better-qualified service staff, increase the retirement contributions, especially for the younger doctors, and pay themselves more. One chairman complained that he was the lowest paid chairman in his specialty in the country.

could reduce what it pays MFA for educational services—about $6 million in 2005—if the practice plan resists the university's bidding.* "Far from what we had hoped, Alan [Wasserman, the MFA chairman] has a very impaired hand to play." Faculty wonder whether this results from a strong negotiating stance taken by the university or a surrender by the MFA leadership to what has been called an "absurd threat," or a combination of the two.

University president Stephen Trachtenberg told the MFA leaders that there had to be a firewall between them and the university and warned, "If you get in trouble, don't come to us." To accomplish this and protect the university from further financial losses, officers of the university could not dominate the board. Accordingly, the doctors on the board serve as members of MFA, which employs them, and not as members of the university faculty.[4]

Despite the separation, says one of the trustees, "We're linked at the hip. The public sees the full-time doctors as GW doctors."[17] Consequently, as one of the veteran clinicians says, "If we really were separate, it might work better, and the firewall would be stronger." Now, the firewall looks decidedly porous.

Operations and Finances

Medical Faculty Associates employs most of the 250 full-time members of the clinical faculty at the George Washington University medical school. A few members of the clinical departments who are primarily investigators remain university employees.[4] According to the affiliation agreement establishing the independent group practice, each of the hospital-based doctors in the clinical laboratories, emergency medicine, pathology, and radiology must be members of MFA.[33]

The clinicians receive one salary check from MFA and none from the university or hospital.[1] The hospital supports the salary of clinicians for the medical administrative work they perform there as well as of those recruited with hospital resources as part of their packages. This money flows from the hospital to MFA, which issues the paychecks. The school does not supplement, with a few exceptions, the salaries paid by MFA to the clinical

---

*The agreement stipulates that, during MFA's first five years, the school could not reduce this amount, but now that restriction no longer applies.

chairmen, division chiefs, and other faculty members for the work they perform directing academic programs.

By 2005, the MFA leaders assert that their enterprise had become the largest multi-specialty group practice in the Washington area with the "best contracts in town," able to extract better rates of as much as 20 percent from the insurers than any other group[34,35] and operating more efficiently than when the university ran it.[4,28,35,36] "It's our business," explains Joseph Giordano, the chairman of surgery. "We decide the issues."[37] The efficient operation of MFA enables what one chairman calls "nimble physician-managers" to succeed at GW. "The average MD now understands better how to make a go of it."[24] Unlike the days when the university was running MFA, "there's much more transparency now," according to Dr. Michael Berrigan, the chairman of anesthesiology and critical care medicine. "One can get any data one wants."[33]

Because it has retained little cash, MFA has no reserve to absorb losses.[33] Accordingly, business management has to be much more efficient than when the university and medical center was there to make up losses. When formed, the practice plan was "just about breaking even," according to Jerry Bass, who had previously been MFA's administrator.[12] People at MFA, however, claim that its deficit was $9 million per year then, and that they have reversed these losses so that MFA has, in recent years, made a small surplus or sustained only a small loss. Accounts receivable have decreased from ninety to fifty-six days, which MFA leaders ascribe to more efficient billing and collecting than was possible by using university facilities.

To maintain solvency, no bonuses are paid unless the corporation can afford it, a significant change from when the practice plan operated under the auspices of the university. Salaries of nonproductive doctors, including some chairmen, have been decreased, an action that produced, not surprisingly, significant unhappiness. "We have to make our salaries," Wasserman explains.[4]

MFA pays the benefits of the doctors, negotiates managed care contracts, and operates the self-insurance trust for its malpractice. The association, which owns no physical property, leases the building where the doctors work from the university on favorable terms[4] of about one-third of the market value, which constitutes, in effect, a subsidy from the medical school.[17] This building is located a city block from the new hospital and the medical school. Some of the doctors also work at facilities associated with GW away from the campus, including two emergency departments that the MFA staffs.

Since separating from the university, MFA operates its own human resources and information technology departments, which the doctors see as
significantly improving the operation.[38] Recently, MFA installed a clinical
information computer system.[39]

Financial support for these improvements requires MFA to tax its clinical
departments in addition to the 3.5 percent external tax required by the
medical school on MFA. The internal tax is theoretically imposed on the
more financially successful departments to support those needing help.
Some chairmen complain that the tax is "set by Badger and Wasserman
with no system but by whim with no input from the chairs," and in some
cases is unfair.[40]

Despite these accomplishments, however, one clinical chairman calls
MFA "a very fragile organization."[33]

Research and Education

MFA does not support its doctors to perform research, for which they
must obtain independent funding.[4]* This means that the clinical departments have difficulty providing start-up funds for young investigators[42]
and helps to explain why the medical school continues to be, when compared with other schools, relatively unproductive in clinical research and
unsuccessful in obtaining research funding. MFA has no central office to
assist investigators in budgeting and in grant writing and management.
Each department must provide these services, and few do. Nor does GW
have an National Institutes of Health (NIH)–supported General Clinical
Research Center (GCRC), "which can be a strong incentive to clinical research," acknowledges one of the clinical chiefs.[25]

The emphasis of MFA being clinical practice—as one chairman put it,
"clinical programs always trump"[43]—there is little time or inclination for
most of the clinical faculty and trainees to perform research.[3,20,27,29,37,41-46]
One basic science chairman suspects that his colleagues in the full-time clinical faculty are "penalized if they do research," because MFA needs money
from clinical practice.[20] Michael Berrigan, who holds a Ph.D. in addition to
his M.D. degree, said, "I would have difficulty recruiting a pure researcher if
he or she did not bring in enough revenue from grants of other sources to

---

*The clinical departments object to their members' not receiving salary bonuses for obtaining
grants as are awarded to members of the basic science departments.[41]

cover his or her expenses."[33] David Reiss, the well-funded investigator in psychiatry, who stayed in the medical school when MFA left, agrees that the current arrangement does not favor the production of clinical research.[47] Only two clinical departments have RO-1 grants from the NIH, although, according to Skip Williams, this represents a recent improvement.[8]

Members of MFA with opinions on the matter believe that separation of the practice plan from the university has not improved this problem[28] and may even have worsened it,[3,41,43,47] an interpretation with which Donald Lehman, the university's executive vice president for academic affairs, agrees. "MFA has no money for it," Lehman, a physicist, says.[48] "The emphasis is now focused on patients in order to meet the bottom line, which means there are not adequate funds or 'release time' to carry out research initiatives."[49]*

Dr. John Kelly, chairman of the department of neurology, who had an active research career before coming to GW, claims he must now devote 80 percent of his time to clinical work because "our money must come out of the department, and our expenses are so high. We must bring in two-and-a-half times what we receive; in a neurology practice, the ratio is closer to one-and-a-half to one. In this climate, it is impossible for me to even consider recruiting someone serious about clinical research."[25] "GW has never emphasized research anyway," one of the clinical chairmen observed.[6]

As for education, the separate practice plan was charged to continue to provide the same quality of services to the students and trainees as when the university owned the practice plan.[17] The consensus is that separation has neither significantly harmed nor improved the clinical teaching programs.

Appointment of Chairmen

Since MFA obtains and processes the clinical income, its trustees and physician leaders can exercise significant influence on the appointment of chairmen of the clinical departments.[24] For example, in the spring of 2005, when the medical school was recruiting a chairman of one of the surgical departments, among the finalists was a clinical investigator with impressive accomplishments in research who would bring several competitive grants

---

*In 2004, the NIH ranked the department of medicine, traditionally the department in medical schools with the largest amount of research activity, 90th of 123 schools (73rd percentile). The department's doctors have 9 NIH grants earning $3,089,097.[50]

with him. One of the other candidates was known primarily as a successful clinician. In addition to the medical school and MFA with an intense interest in recruitments at this level was the hospital, whose leaders are charged to keep the beds full of paying patients. The clinician had a greater appeal to them than the researcher, and he was offered the job.

This was not the first time that such a controversy occurred. When the chairmanship of another surgical specialty opened, the hospital and the voluntary faculty successfully lobbied the dean to promote the acting chairman, who had a large practice but was not his first choice on academic grounds.

In January 2006, Alan Wasserman told the clinical departments that all future clinical chairmen must be appointed from within GW since MFA could not afford any more external searches. The stimulus for this action was the recent recruitment of Dr. Thomas Jarrett from Johns Hopkins, who, after three searches had failed to fill the chair, became the first permanent chairman of urology since 1995. Jarrett, as in the case of several faculty members recruited from other institutions, had a strong connection to Washington. His first faculty position after training was at GW, and for the nine subsequent years that he was a member of the Hopkins faculty, he and his family continued to live in Chevy Chase, a Washington suburb. So Jarrett was glad to work again in Washington, D.C., bring his special skills in noninvasive surgery on the kidney to GW, and, not totally incidentally, reduce his commute. Jarrett's patients from the Washington area—30 to 40 percent of his practice at Hopkins—will now see him at GW.[5]

The medical school, MFA, and Universal wanted Jarrett for his clinical skills and, anticipating sizeable financial returns, were prepared to invest significant resources in his appointment. It was the combination of the hospital and the medical school—particularly dean James Scott—who convinced him to move. As for MFA, Jarrett says, "I would have been turned off if they were the only entity [trying to recruit me]."[5] Particularly troubling to Jarrett were the benefits MFA provided, or more relevant, did not provide. Jarrett would lose the tuition benefit for his children that Hopkins grants and would not be able to participate in the MFA retirement plan until he had been there for five years. Whether MFA would permit a sabbatical, Jarrett could not determine.[5]*

*One of the clinical chairs says, "You can take a sabbatical but neither the university nor MFA provides any funds. You have to get the funding yourself. So, for most, there is no sabbatical,"[51] providing another disincentive to perform research, which is why few clinical faculty members take sabbaticals.

Wasserman's announcement confirmed what had become the pattern at GW. Not directing resources to recruit chairmen, who could bring strong programs from other schools,[24,30] helps to explain why most of the current clinical chairmen were members of the GW faculty when appointed and why some of the departments have been led by acting or interim chairmen for many years. Accordingly, faculty members describe the clinical departments as having "a great deal of inbreeding."

Voluntary Faculty; Town-Gown Issues

GW has long depended on its voluntary faculty to help teach the students and trainees and fill the beds at the University Hospital.[52] Many, if not most, are alumni of the GW medical school or one of its training programs for residents and fellows. Some are leading private practitioners in Washington. Most receive no money from the university and support themselves with their private practices.[47]

Although valuing the contributions of the voluntary faculty, "the institution had little control over the teaching performed by them," remembers Lloyd Elliott, president of the university from 1965 to 1988. "The dean was quite frustrated by this."[9] Responding to this problem and to pressure from hospital licensing authorities officials, the school started, by the 1970s, to appoint doctors to full-time positions in the clinical departments.[9] GW began this process so late, however, that it became one of the last of the older medical schools to do so.[53]

Gradually, full-time faculty came to dominate the clinical departments so that, within a decade, their patients filled many, though not a majority, of the beds in the hospital. Most of the doctors recruited for these positions emphasized clinical care and teaching in their work, as had their voluntary brethren, and not research. Over the years, this pattern has continued. As Philip Birnbaum, a longtime senior administrator at the medical center, observed, "These doctors tended to replicate themselves."[54]

Conflict between the voluntary and full-time faculty has been long-standing, with the voluntary faculty accusing the full-timers of inefficient operations compared with the way they run their private practices.[55] The local practitioners were "very irritated, a classic town-gown problem," in the words of Dr. Dennis O'Leary, an early member of the full-time faculty and, during his fifteen-year career at GW, vice president of the health plan and medical director of the University Hospital.* "Our problems became nationally known," O'Leary remembers, "what with the District of Columbia Medical Society just down the block."[53]

"The place had thrived for years on its voluntary faculty," observed Dr. Stephen Schimpff from the University of Maryland when he looked at the position of vice president for medical affairs at GW in 1993.[56] Schimpff saw that some of the full-time doctors were "making life bad" for the voluntary faculty, who for years had been the "heart and soul" of GW. He heard that many were taking their practices to other hospitals partly because the facilities in the old university hospital were so unappealing to private patients and partly because the full-time staff made practice there so difficult.[56]

"When I got there," remembers Dan McLean, the former CEO of the hospital, "I found a feeling that some of the full-time chiefs wanted the voluntary medical staff to disappear despite their value to the hospital." McLean felt that some of the full-time faculty were acting as if they believed that "it's our playground. Stay away."[57] As the hospital director, McLean believed that this attitude made no sense because the voluntary faculty medical staff were admitting 60 percent of the patients to the hospital.[57]

Full-Time versus Voluntary Faculty in Cardiology and Cardiac Surgery

Despite the building of the new university hospital and a deliberate effort by the clinical and hospital leadership recently to attract voluntary physicians, "town-gown conflicts are remembered to this second," said Dr. Richard Katz, the chief of cardiology. "We're still angry with you because you wouldn't open the [cardiac catheterization] lab to us," he has heard voluntary cardiologists tell him even now.[34] Because of this policy and the decrepit state of the old hospital, cardiologists with GW appointments took many of their patients to other hospitals, particularly the Washington Hospital Center, where they could perform the procedures themselves.[58] They then kept their patients who needed cardiac surgery there, where the service was seen as superior to that available at GW.[58]

Allowing only full-time cardiologists to work in the university hospital

---

*On leaving GW in 1986, O'Leary became president of the Joint Commission on Accreditation of Healthcare Organizations in Oakbrook Terrace, Illinois.

catheterization laboratory had long been the custom not only at GW but at most academic medical centers. However, decreasing numbers of patients and the income their care generates were forcing hospital and physician leaders to open their labs to voluntary faculty and allow them to treat their patients there. Hospital executives realized that more patients being studied in their laboratories would result in more patients having other tests performed at the hospital and more patients having their operations performed there. These patients would also present the clinicians with more patients who needed consultations.

In the mid-1990s, Dr. Roger Meyer, during his brief tenure as vice president for medical affairs, had opened the labs[59] over the objections of some of the full-time doctors.[34] The chief of cardiology at the time "wouldn't even let practicing cardiologists come and train in our labs," the current chief remembered. "This caused much hard feelings."[34] It was not until the new University Hospital opened in 2002 that the voluntary cardiologists began to bring their patients there in relatively large numbers. When the lab was closed, the full-time faculty performed less than a thousand procedures a year. With the lab open to community cardiologists, the number of procedures rose to 2,500 per year, with the voluntary faculty doing about three-quarters of the cases.

One of these voluntary cardiologists is Dr. Joel Rosenberg, who used to care for his patients at the Washington Hospital Center "even though we wanted to go with GW, which was downtown much nearer our offices." Now, he is working almost exclusively at GW because of the efforts of the hospital administration, not the MFA. "Four years ago, the CEO [of the GW hospital, now under Universal ownership] approached me to become clinical director of cardiology, a parallel path with MFA. I would focus on the clinical effort and Richard Katz on the academic side."[58]

It was the hospital, not the medical school or MFA, that contracted with Rosenberg for this service. "The hospital wanted additional leadership. It needed patients and programs, and the full-timers weren't providing them," Rosenberg explains. "They didn't respond to the hospital's need for new ideas and a better connection with the private sector. The transition was difficult for Dick [Katz] and the MFA leadership,"[58] but they could not effectively object because the hospital was now owned by Universal and no longer by the medical school. Rosenberg asks, "If voluntary cardiologists could have used the cath lab and voluntary cardiac surgeons had been more welcome at GW years ago, would the hospital have had to be sold?"[58]

Rosenberg then describes the problems he and his colleagues see with full-time clinical doctors. "We're out there in the trenches drumming up patients. The full-timers are waiting for the patients to come to them. I've seen this from a twenty-year perspective at GW."[58]

The difficulties in medical cardiology extended to the cardiac surgical service.[19,60] "The old policy of prohibiting voluntary faculty from using the cath lab had a long-term negative effect on cardiology and cardiac surgery that even today influences cardiac surgery," says surgery chairman Joseph Giordano, who has tried and consistently failed to recruit a full-time cardiac surgeon who could succeed at GW. "I won't hire another," he said in the spring of 2005. "We lost money on each of them, got burned too often. Let the private groups do it."[37]

And that is what has happened. An example is Dr. Nevin Katz, who joined George Washington and MFA in 2001 soon after the practice plan at Georgetown was sold to MedStar. "We wanted to set up an institute within GW," Katz says, "but despite many discussions it didn't work out. It has not been clear to me why, as the minimally invasive surgery of the new institute seemed to fit well at GW. Perhaps the MFA leadership thought the institute structure would give us too much independence."[61] So Katz and four of his surgical colleagues left the full-time faculty and established the Washington Institute of Thoracic and Cardiovascular Surgery on K Street near the GW University Hospital, where they admit many of their patients. MFA sued the surgeons of the institute for violating noncompete clauses, "but we worked out a favorable settlement."[61] Nevin Katz now directs the institute's cardiothoracic critical care unit.*

Another cardiac surgeon who left MFA and later the full-time faculty in Giordano's department is Dr. Mark Adkins, who operated at GW from 1999 to 2004. Not long after he arrived, Adkins was distressed to learn that many

---

*Nevin Katz trained at highly respected institutions: B.A., Swarthmore; M.D., Case (Alpha Omega Alpha,); general surgical and cardiothoracic surgical training at the Massachusetts General and Children's hospitals in Boston and at the University of Alabama. Katz's title is clinical professor of surgery. At GW and at many medical schools the prefix "clinical" in the academic title indicates that the physician is not a full-time employee of the medical school or, at GW, of MFA.

of the promises made by the school and MFA during the recruitment process would not be fulfilled due to lack of funds. Then, one year later, Adkins
"found on my desk a new contract from MFA," which had just separated
from the university. Not liking some of its provisions, Adkins decided to remain an employee of the university, the only full-time clinician at the time
to do so.[62]

When his three-year contract with the university ended, Adkins left the
full-time faculty and opened an office across the street from the hospital,
continued to operate there, and held the title of clinical director of cardiac
surgery. In 2004, he left GW for a professorship at the Weill Medical College
of Cornell University in New York City.

The GW hospital needed a cardiac surgeon to replace Adkins and, de-
spairing that the medical school and MFA could recruit one, the hospital
director hired his own team.* The new chief of cardiac surgery, Dr. Frederick
Lough, and his colleague Dr. Farzad Najam, who had been practicing privately and operating at the George Washington University Hospital, became the first full-time doctors reporting to the CEO and paid by the hospital. They would not be members of MFA but would report for academic
matters to the chairman of the department of surgery in the medical school,
Joseph Giordano. "I was very comfortable with this arrangement," said
Lough, "given that I have known Joe for thirty years."[63]

One reason Lough chose this administrative arrangement is that, if he
joined MFA, he was told by several people, few of the voluntary physicians
would refer him patients.[63] In recognition of his participation in the teaching of medical students and trainees, the school appointed him clinical
professor of surgery.

Frederick Lough, like his friend Mark Adkins, had grown up in the Washington area. He attended West Point, as had his father and now his son.
Deciding to become a doctor, Lough entered the class of 1975 at GW, where
Paul Adkins, the chairman of surgery and Mark's father, strongly influenced
him to become a cardiac surgeon. After graduating first in his class, training
in his specialty, and fulfilling his obligation to the army, Lough practiced
cardiac surgery in Pennsylvania and Texas. He resumed his affiliation with

---

*According to the terms under which MFA was established, the practice plan has the right of
"first refusal." Only if MFA cannot or does not want to hire a physician or surgeon that the hospital
needs can the hospital do so on its own.[1]

GW in 2005 and not before then, he says, because of "a continuation of long-term stumbling" in the development of medical and surgical cardiology. "History shadows everything," he adds.[63]

Thus, a private company, Universal Health Services, Inc., which owns 80 percent of the George Washington University Hospital, now employs its own doctors there, although the company has always resisted doing so at its other hospitals. "We will do what we have to do from the business perspective in spite of our relation with the MFA," explains Dr. Carlos Silva, the hospital medical director.[35]*

Other Departments

Access to patients coming to the University Hospital emergency department without a doctor of their own long produced conflict between full-time and voluntary faculty. Until the rules in force when the university owned the hospital were recently changed, all such patients were assigned to the full-time faculty and could account for a significant part of these doctors' practices. Voluntary cardiologists who wanted to accept patients from the emergency department were not welcome there.

Under Universal, the hospital pressed the full-time clinicians to allow several private cardiologists to participate in the cardiology emergency department on-call schedule. Richard Katz remembers that the battle with the hospital over this issue was "the biggest fight we had, sending me to the mat. We argued that doing so for one doctor would set a bad precedent."[34] The full-timers compromised and assigned the doctor to the emergency department on Mondays from 7:00 a.m. to 7:00 p.m.[34] "Of course, he has to offer follow-up care to uninsured as well as insured patients coming there," observed Katz with a glimmer of satisfaction.[34] Since the rule was changed, a second internist on the voluntary staff was permitted to participate, joining doctors from other departments with these privileges.

The hospital executives have appointed some of the voluntary faculty to newly created positions as clinical or co-directors of several of the busier clinical services and laboratories and pay them part-time salaries for the

---

*The hospital bills for Lough's and Najam's professional services and pays them salaries with incentives if they exceed certain levels of activity.[64]

administrative work they perform for the hospital.* The amount of money paid to all the voluntary faculty—about $1.5 million per year, according to Skip Williams's office—compares with the hospital's support of $4 million to MFA for work performed by the full-time faculty.[8] The hospital pays some of the voluntary faculty to co-administer some of the clinical services and is paying more attention than in the past to other wishes of the voluntary faculty. "They have other places to go," as one of the clinical chairmen observed, "unlike us [full-time doctors] who usually work only at University Hospital."[28]

In a recent change of potentially significant importance, the hospital, to increase admissions, has begun to invite physicians and surgeons to admit their patients without requiring participation in the teaching programs traditionally expected of all who admit to teaching hospitals.

Town-Gown Relationships Improve

The town-gown conflicts may be decreasing, according to Joel Rosenberg, the director of clinical cardiology. "The level of paranoia is less, but there are still problems."[58] Most doctors in each group send their patients to their own type of doctor, the full-timers usually referring within MFA and the voluntary faculty to other voluntary faculty. The voluntary faculty complain that they lose the income generated by tests† on patients they admit to the hospital since the hospital and MFA perform these procedures and the full-time doctors interpret the results.

"Despite bringing patients to GW, we're still not fully accepted," Rosenberg says. "The hospital benefits from the work of the voluntary doctors, who provide new and alternative ways to care for patients and new ideas that may not already exist in the more closed and inbred environment of a full-time system. MFA doesn't appreciate the dollars we send their way." Rosenberg feels that MFA should be "more inclusive in policy making. They should be more proactive, invite us in, and thank us for the teaching we do and the business we provide."[58]

To attract more voluntary faculty into closer association with the full-

---

*Some of the full-time doctors see these appointments as an effort by the hospital administration to please the voluntary faculty and attract them to admit their patients to University Hospital.[22,28,34]

†Called "downstream revenue."

timers—"bring them into our tent," as one of the practice plan executives explained—Medical Faculty Associates offers to assume some of the administrative burden that all but the largest groups find difficult to perform efficiently and economically. Among these services are billing and collecting of fees, contracting for managed care contracts, and supporting computer technology. MFA benefits by charging fees for these services, thereby decreasing its average overhead through the greater size of the services it administers. Relieved of these administrative hassles, the voluntary faculty then cover the other costs of their practices and their salaries from the proceeds MFA sends them. The system makes some money for MFA and links its members more closely to the practitioners. Such a new business initiative would not have been possible, the MFA leaders believe, when the practice plan was part of the university with its risk-adverse philosophy.

Some of the clinical chairs also believe that town-gown dealings have improved. "Our relationship with the voluntary faculty is not a problem," says surgery chair Joseph Giordano, "because I understand where they're coming from."[37] His department has fifteen full-time faculty members, but about 40 percent of the surgeons who practice at University Hospital are voluntary faculty.[37]

One of them used to be Dr. Carlos Silva, a member of the GW class of 1960. After taking his residency at the GW hospital, Silva set up a private practice of general surgery with a particular interest in patients with burns in downtown Washington and admitted his patients to several hospitals, including GW. When Silva stopped accepting insurance because of the administrative and financial hassles associated with it, the number of operations he performed fell from about sixty to fifteen per week. The income of his practice, however, did not drop significantly—he was able to collect more money per case than when he accepted insurance—but when his overhead started rising, the practice began to lose money. "I was working too hard for not enough money," he said.[35]

So in 2003, Silva joined MFA. With the administration of his practice, including his malpractice insurance, taken on more economically by the group practice, which accepted insurance, and with the better rates MFA could obtain from the insurers, Silva's income returned to its former level. Two years later, when Silva started thinking about retiring from practice, the hospital asked him to become its medical director. Now he is a full-time administrator with an office in the hospital. He reports to both the hospital director and the dean. His paycheck comes from the school of medicine, but the hospital supports 60 percent[12] of it. MFA transferred the care of his patients to other members of the group.[35]

Dr. David Simon, a general internist, is another longtime private practitioner who recently became full-time and joined MFA. "Though I took a 15 percent pay cut, it was worth it. I enjoy teaching and can now do more of it. I see fewer patients than when I was in practice, and night call is certainly easier. One's day work is more spread out in practice, more compressed here." But working for MFA is not perfect. "Compared with private practice, MFA's cumbersome. There's more inertia. The good thing is that you work for a big bureaucracy. The bad thing is that you work for a big bureaucracy."[65]

With an attractive new hospital, the GW voluntary faculty who had been admitting their patients to other hospitals are returning. They appreciate that management is according them greater visibility[31] and respect—though not enough for some[58]—than in the past.

Was Separation Wise?

Among MFA's more outspoken critics are former chairmen of clinical departments and other faculty members who have left the university.

- "Those chairmen who, like me, favored change were outvoted by the others. Some were protecting special deals they had made with favorites."
- "GW used to be a great place known for several [clinical] departments. I noted in the recent *U.S. News & World Report* listing that GW did not make the top hundred in any category."
- "There's much dead wood among the chairs and division heads. They think they're academic leaders—though most of them are not—and rather than go out and develop practices, they sit around and politic and assume that patients will come to them because they're professors. As for the young people, they work them to death and pay them badly, so many leave."*

---

*Readers should bear in mind that although some of these comments may describe real deficiencies, others may reflect ill feelings related to the circumstances under which the faculty member left, or was forced to leave, GW and MFA.

Other observers are more positive about the independent practice plan. "Separating MFA from the university was good," says former hospital CEO Dan McLean. "It really does make the doctors responsible and emphasizes that production is important."[57] McLean believes, however, that the members of MFA "are still leveraged against the community doctors. Nevertheless, it's a cleaner, meaner machine than it was."[57]

University executive vice president Louis Katz remembers that before MFA became independent, "there was much more finger-pointing, accountability was poor, and it wasn't all that entrepreneurial. Now that they're responsible, it's improved. The docs work harder and better."[2] Asked how the clinical faculty would react if the medical school tried to regain full control of the practice plan, Katz replied, "They'd be very unhappy, but less so if we gave them some capital."[2] Skip Williams would "like to have them back, but there'll be headaches whether they're in or out."[8]

Robert Perry, the trustee who chairs the medical committee of the board, observes that "creating MFA was a high-risk proposition. It's too soon to say if the separate practice plan will be a successful model. We've had trials and tribulations, but I'm optimistic."[17] Perry points to the favorable financial results, the growing responsibility that the doctors are taking for the plan's performance, and the new information technology system as evidence that MFA is making progress. "If we hadn't done it, we'd have other and possibly worse problems."[17]

CHAPTER FOUR

George Washington University

Closing the HMO

In 1970, Dr. Thomas Piemme came to GW from the University of Pittsburgh to direct all ambulatory programs that were not part of the private practices of the faculty. His responsibilities included running the emergency department as well as the clinics. Piemme's interests included prepaid health plans, and he proceeded to establish the second health maintenance organization (HMO) in the district.[1] GW's HMO was unique in having been started just before the federal HMO law was enacted.[2]

"Our HMO and the department of health care sciences [its related academic department in the medical center] was clearly ahead of their time," said Dr. Gregory Pawlson, who would chair the department from 1987 to 1998 after the HMO had been split off as a separate entity.[3] In the 1970s, few at GW had an interest in primary care. The chairman of the department of medicine at the time actively opposed the effort.

The first members of the HMO were Medicaid patients, although not those in the GW clinics.[1] Before the HMO, university hospital clinics were not the most inviting places for patients to attend. The patients did not receive specific appointments and often had to wait for hours before being seen. Their doctor was usually an intern or resident with medical students actively participating. The amount of supervision they received from members of the faculty was variable. Piemme and his colleagues, who were assigned the management of the clinics, gave each patient a specific appointment. A member of his group saw or supervised the care of each of them. When the HMO started, the hospital clinics serving Medicaid patients were closed, saving $500,000 per year for the university hospital.[4]

The university president at the time, who originally favored the HMO being established as part of the university, was convinced to allow the unit to be incorporated separately. Even so, doctors and officials from GW dominated the board of directors. Among the doctors who worked in the HMO some were physicians on short-term appointments at the nearby National Institutes of Health (NIH) in Bethesda who wanted to continue seeing patients as primary care physicians to supplement the research they were performing at the NIH.[1]

The HMO Prospers

In 1974, the medical school decided to create a separate "department of health care sciences" for all the primary care programs at GW, which would be separate from, but equal to, the department of medicine where Piemme and his group were initially assigned. "I wanted to call it the 'department of primary care,'" Piemme remembers.[1]* The school began a search for a chairman of the new department of health care sciences. Although Piemme was one of the leading candidates, he was not chosen.†

The doctor selected for the job was Dr. John Ott from the University of Colorado,[2,3] who remembers, "When I arrived at GW in 1977, the health plan had about seven thousand members, essentially all of whom were transfers from the clinic."[4] With a health plan, a primary care network, a wholly owned hospital, and a clinical faculty of full-time and voluntary faculty, GW had developed what one of the hospital administrators called "one of the first truly integrated delivery systems."[6]

Gradually, the HMO grew to about a hundred thousand subscribers.

---

*In 2006, GW was one of the few U.S. medical schools without a department or program of family medicine.[5]

†Piemme became director and then associate dean of GW's office of continuing education from 1979 until he retired from the university in 1998.

While the HMO initially used only the university's full-time faculty for both primary and specialty care, conflicts arose over relatively restrictive payments to specialists and the hospital and the need for primary care referrals.[7-9] Eventually, the HMO's patients accounted for about 20 percent of all the admissions to the George Washington University Hospital. In some specialties, the HMO contributed as many as one-third of the patients to the practices.

The HMO provided important contributions to GW's educational and research missions, with students and trainees working in its multi-specialty primary care group practice.[2,10,11] With the number of patients in the plan growing, more became well-insured federal employees.[10]

Selling and Buying Back the HMO

Despite its demonstrated value to education and as a source of primary care patients for the specialists on the faculty, the university sold the HMO to a large for-profit hospital corporation in 1985 in anticipation of selling the GW hospital to the same corporation.[12,13] University executives had become convinced that the HMO needed between two hundred thousand and three hundred thousand subscribers to be successful and did not want to spend the money required to recruit the additional subscribers.[2] In the next year-and-a-half, the corporation lost $10 million on the HMO.[2] So the company sold the health plan back to GW for between $9 and $10 million; the company had paid $13 million to purchase it less than two years previously.[2] The company had failed to make a success of the HMO because, as two GW medical officials said, "they had no experience, didn't know what they were getting into," and "the for-profits don't know how to do non-profit business."

"We salvaged it," said Ott.[2] Within a year after GW had reacquired the health plan, it became profitable, with surpluses of as much as $7 million annually for several years. This allowed the HMO to accumulate a reserve of $30 million, which it needed to function successfully as an insurance company. The cash flow from the HMO assured the medical center's solvency, according to Ott.[2]

The HMO had, at its beginning, paid the university more than what the market required for primary care services, a form of subsidy to the medical school and faculty practices that paid the doctors' salaries. The GW special-

ists, both full-time and voluntary, however, maintained that they were receiving less than the market would have paid them for patients referred
through the HMO.[7,14,15] "Actually," according to Dr. Thompson Bowles,
executive vice president of the medical center from 1987 to 1992, "they
were facing what all payers were doing, and they didn't like it."[7]

By 1995, the insurance cycle and competition among health plans caused
the HMO to lose $1.5 million[8] on an operating basis of $140 million, and Ott
was fired as director of the HMO. He negotiated a settlement and retired as
an emeritus professor.[2]

GW hired the Hunter Group, a consulting firm that specialized in helping academic medical centers with financial problems, to manage the plan
and try to improve its finances. As Ott saw the situation, the HMO lost
increasingly more money, and many patients left.[2] According to one of the
division chiefs, doctors left as well, some going to Georgetown.[9] Conversion to a for-profit venture would have been expensive because the district's
laws would have required that the university pay a sizeable tax for the
change.[11]

The university, which had vacillated about keeping, selling, or closing
the plan, decided, in 1998, to try to make it work again[16] and recruited
Stanley Aronovitch, an experienced health care executive, as CEO.[17] For a
while under its new CEO, the plan prospered, but by 2000, it was struggling
again as competition increased. "We had 85,000 to 90,000 members, not
enough to be effective," Aronovitch remembers. "Provider-sponsored plans
like ours were failing."[17]

One of the purposes of GW's HMO was to supply referrals to the hospital
and to the full-time doctors, paying them fees that were higher than the
market demanded.* "A big reason that the HMO was losing money," a consultant concluded, "was because it was required to subsidize MFA, which
should have had to operate on its own bottom line."

When the university separated from its practice plan, Medical Faculty
Associates closed some of the community practice sites, complicating the
marketing of the HMO. Furthermore, stories in the newspapers that GW
might dispose of the HMO did not encourage new members to join. Meanwhile, selling the HMO as one of the options also became increasingly
difficult. Managed care companies were not attracted to a plan without a

---

*One of the trustees called the HMO "a funneling system."[18]

substantial primary care practice that referred its patients to high-charging university specialists and their expensive hospital.[1,17,19] Seeing no productive future in his position, Aronovitch left GW and its HMO three years after arriving.[17]*

Closing the HMO

In 2002, with the HMO continuing to lose money and the value of HMOs like GW's falling, the university decided to close the plan.[20] Despite its value in referring patients to the full-time faculty and the hospital, the HMO was never a favorite arm of the university, whose executives were not unhappy about closing it. Some felt that, as "a small boutique health plan,"[21] it was too small to ever succeed.[22,23] Furthermore, observes Dr. Sheldon Retchin, vice president for health sciences at Virginia Commonwealth University and CEO of the VCU Health System,† which includes a large, successful HMO, "they never work as a feeder."[24]

Ott blames the fate of the HMO on the university's risk-adverse philosophy, which was inconsistent with running a health plan. "You can't be risk-adverse in the insurance business," Ott felt. "I believe that the HMO could have succeeded. Getting rid of it was imprudent."[2]‡

Michael Barch, the former hospital CEO, estimated that closing the HMO cost the university $13 million. "They could have given it away and saved money," he said.[10] "Actually," says Gregory Pawlson, "the HMO could likely have been sold in the early 1990s,"[3] when it still had value in the market.§ As Louis Katz observed, "We waited too long."[25]

---

*After leaving GW, Aronovitch became president and CEO of the Mercy Care Plan in Phoenix, Arizona.[17]

†And at one time a candidate for the vice presidency at GW.

‡Gregory Pawlson observed, "While Jack Ott did bring the HMO back to some stability, the lack of support on the part of the university to his attempt to grow market share by low balling the premium and aggressive marketing doomed both the plan and Dr. Ott's tenure at GW."[13]

§Selling is what the trustees had intended in the 1980s when they sold, but then took back, the plan from the for-profit company.

CHAPTER FIVE

George Washington University and Its Medical School

Because it would be located in the federal city and not in a state, it was the U.S. Congress that created "The Columbian College in the District of Columbia," and it was President James Monroe who approved its establishment on February 9, 1821.* The founder of the university, Reverend Luther Price, a Baptist minister, wanted the General Convention of the Baptist Denomination in the United States to take a leading role in its administration, but Congress refused to accept this church-state arrangement and decreed that all religious tests be prohibited.

Although part of the original plans of Columbian College, its medical school did not open until March 1825, four years after the founding of the college. Of the 126 medical schools in the United States in 2006, the George Washington University School of Medicine—the college had become Columbian University in 1873 and George Washington University in 1904—is the twelfth oldest.[3]

---

*This history of the university, medical school, and hospital has been adapted from the books by Elmer Louis Kayser.[1,2]

The medical school, like many in the nineteenth century, was propri-
etary, owned by the doctors on the faculty, who assumed all risks and operated autonomously and independent of the college. The relationship between the college and what was then called its "Medical Department" was
slight and formal, limited to the conferring of degrees and approval of
faculty nominated by the school, and so it remained for many years. There
were six students in the first and eight in the second graduating classes,
a size that continued for several years. The students were taught in the
school's first building, erected by the doctors at Tenth and E streets.

In 1844, the school—in effect, its faculty—assumed ownership of the
Washington Infirmary, originally a jail, then an insane asylum, and eventually a general hospital "for the sick and the treatment of paupers" and
located on Judiciary Square at Fifth and F streets. Congress had not assigned
the infirmary to the college but rather to the medical faculty, which equipped,
maintained, and improved it. The city assumed some responsibility for the
financial support of the patients. At the beginning of the Civil War in 1861,
the federal government requisitioned the infirmary but could only use it
for a short time because the building was destroyed by fire in November of
that year.

The medical school also suffered from the effects of the war as personnel
and students joined the armies, and it was forced to conduct its business in
several different buildings until 1866. In that year, thanks to a gift to Columbian College from William Wilson Corcoran (1798–1888),* the school
moved into a handsome new building on the north side of H Street between
Thirteenth and Fourteenth streets, where, if one includes a replacement, it
would remain for a century. The custom continued whereby any income
remaining after paying the expenses of operating the college was divided
among the faculty.

By 1877, the curriculum, revised to include a graded course and regular
examinations, was beginning to approach the instructional system still
used today. The basic sciences—"the seven essential branches of medical
science," according to the school's catalogue at the time—were taught in
the first two years and the clinical courses in the third year, although some
clinics were held in the second year. Students continued to buy tickets from

---

*Founder of the Corcoran Gallery of Art, for nearly fifty years after its founding in 1874 the only
art museum in Washington.[4,5]

the professors to attend their lectures and demonstrations. The courses leading to the M.D. degree cost about $135, but when it was learned that of 63 medical schools, only 18 charged more than $100 and 45 charged less, the fee was dropped to $100. By this time, between 50 and 60 students registered each year. By 1891, the catalogue shows the number to have grown to 158. Eventually, the school increased the course to 4 years, and the ticketing system to attend lectures was discontinued. In 1884, the medical school admitted its first women students, but the faculty revoked this policy in 1892. Twenty years passed before women were readmitted, and this time for good.

Then in 1910 came the Flexner Report. Its review of GW's medical school was brief but scathing.[6]

- Entrance requirements: less than a four-year high school course.
- Teaching staff: other than for three instructors "of other grade," none of the faculty are full-time teachers.
- Resources: GW "lacks adequate resources as well as assured prospects."
- General: GW and Georgetown "are surrounded by medical schools—those of Richmond, Baltimore, Philadelphia—whose competition they cannot meet. . . . Should the District require, as it aught, a higher basis, or even enforce an actual four-year high school standard, both would suffer seriously. Neither school is now equal to the task of training physicians of modern type."

Founding the University Hospital

By 1897, the university trustees had decided to convert into a small hospital the Columbian Academy, a secondary school then being closed, on the north side of H Street east of Fourteenth Street near the medical school. After acquiring adjacent property in 1903, the university built a newer hospital of a hundred beds to replace the short-lived one in the defunct secondary school, which, connected to the new hospital, became a dispensary.* The university also built in the same block a new home for the medical school, which would operate there for the next seventy years. "This hospital was very small," remembers medical school alumnus Dr. Luther

---

*Dispensary—the older term for an outpatient or ambulatory care facility.

Brady, a distinguished radiation oncologist and emeritus GW trustee, "so we took our clinical rotations at what became the DC General Hospital and not at the university hospital."[7]

Finding itself squeezed from having used all the space in the H Street location, the university decided to build a new hospital in the part of the city known as "Foggy Bottom."* In time, the medical school would follow the hospital. Much of the rest of the university, once scattered throughout the district, had begun moving there from the beginning of the century.

The federal government agreed to pay for a hospital with five hundred to six hundred beds in the block between Twenty-second and Twenty-third streets and I ("Eye") Street and Pennsylvania Avenue. Since the government was not obliged to equip the building, the $800,000 required for this purpose was raised privately. Major General U. S. Grant III (retired), the grandson of the eighteenth president and a trustee of the university, led the effort. The new hospital, which opened on March 1, 1948, was called "the most contemporary hospital"[7] in Washington at the time and was described as "six stories in height, limestone-faced, and of reinforced concrete construction; it contained 950 service and patients' rooms. One of the city's largest private buildings, the aggregate floor space of its corridors was said to be equivalent to the street and sidewalk space of seven city blocks."[9]

In 1962, Congress allotted up to $2.5 million, on a matching basis, to expand the hospital. The university proceeded to raise $5.8 million toward the building of the Eugene Meyer Pavilion, which opened four years later. The full capacity of the hospital was now 540 beds. The outpatient clinic (successor to the old dispensary) was moved from the hospital to a new thirteen-story building on the southeast corner of Pennsylvania Avenue and Twenty-second Street.

The basic science departments remained in their downtown location until Ross Hall, the current medical school building, opened in 1973. The growing full-time clinical faculty saw their patients in a nearby converted apartment building that was owned by the university and managed by the hospital.[10]

---

*Foggy Bottom was formerly "bottom land, and much of its lower fringe was swampy," writes university historian Kayser.[8] "The fogs which settled over the river bank were amplified by the smog from the gas works which emitted dirt-laden and malodorous clouds of smoke, day and night, touched up with violent spurts of flame that lit up the vicinity with an eerie glow." That was then. When the university moved there, the gas works were gone, and "in its present fine attire Foggy Bottom has taken on the ways of gentility."[8]

Until the medical school built Ross Hall across I Street from the hospital, the students spent most of their first two years in the old and what has been described as "pretty shabby"[11] facilities on H Street and then moved to the University Hospital in Foggy Bottom and other training sites for the last two years. Luther Brady remembers the old medical school as a "nineteenth-century building where the one elevator was reserved for the faculty." The students had to climb to the top floor for their 8:00 a.m. anatomy lectures. The doors were locked when the lectures began, and each student sat in his or her numbered seat. "Our professor was very Prussian. He insisted that we take all our notes on 5 by 8 cards."[7]*

Accordingly, the basic scientists were geographically separated from the clinical faculty for twenty-five years, which some at the school suggest contributed to the disappointing development of research during that period. Skip Williams suggests that when one considers the accomplishments and reputation of the George Washington University medical school, one should start counting from the opening of Ross Hall in 1973 and not 180 years ago, when the school was founded.[12]

Vice President for Medical Affairs

In 1993, GW needed a new leader of the medical center. One of the candidates who looked at the job was Dr. Stephen Schimpff, then executive vice president at the University of Maryland Medical System in Baltimore. "I found a fairly demoralized institution with minimal research," he remembers.[13] "The place was a mess financially. Neither the hospital nor the school had financial statements." The university, "starting with Trachtenberg," saw the medical center as a burden rather than an opportunity. "It was a cultural thing," Schimpff concluded.[13]

Continuing with the recruitment, Schimpff met some of the leading trustees and concluded that they "weren't paying much attention to the medical center or at least did not appreciate that it was a major element of the university, certainly a very large portion of the total finances." With all that he saw that had to be done, Schimpff anticipated great difficulty "fighting up as well as down and across."[13]

---

*This teacher was a fairly talented musician and kept a piano in the lecture room. Students in labs on other floors could hear him practicing during the day.[7]

Though the search committee and Schimpff thought that he was being hired, at least in part, to fix the hospital, Trachtenberg said to Schimpff after a committee meeting, "I don't know why we don't just sell the hospital." Schimpff concluded that Trachtenberg had already decided to get rid of the hospital. Since running a university hospital is what Schimpff had been doing at Maryland and what he wanted to continue to do for at least part of any new job, he rejected GW when Trachtenberg offered him the job soon afterwards.[13]

The man who took the job was Dr. Roger Meyer, a psychiatrist and Harvard Medical School graduate who had particular interest in the problems of addiction. Meyer's wife and Trachtenberg's wife had become friends in the Hartford area when Trachtenberg was president of the University of Hartford and Meyer was at the University of Connecticut as chairman of psychiatry and later executive dean.

When Meyer started looking at the position at GW, "I went there cautiously," but, to his surprise, Meyer found that he was beginning to like the place and the medical faculty whom he met at GW. "They were like Rodney Dangerfield—no respect but hoping for something better."[14] Trachtenberg offered Meyer the job, and, after a follow-up visit, he accepted the position. In 1993, Meyer became GW's vice president for medical affairs, executive dean, and Walter Bloedorn Professor of Administrative Medicine and professor of psychiatry.

Meyer found an institution with major problems. "It was in receivership," he remembers. "Billing and collecting by the university were lousy; we were even billing Medicare less than Medicare would pay." Meyer brought in a financial consultant from Connecticut, "and we collected $30 million in eighteen months." He also hired Thomas Chapman, an experienced executive who had led other Washington hospitals, as CEO of the George Washington University Hospital. Chapman put together, what Meyer calls, "a great team."[14]

One of Meyer's decisions was to permit voluntary faculty to treat patients in the cardiac catheterization laboratories, where previously only full-time members had privileges. Expectedly, this met with resistance from what he calls "the old guard" clinical leadership.[15]

Meyer and his colleagues wrote a strategic plan that the trustees endorsed, but, according to Meyer, "Steve and Lou Katz blocked it."[15] "Lou was Roger's big problem," an observer said. "He just didn't want to be in the health care business, especially as a provider of medical services." Trachtenberg trusted Katz and depended on him to manage the university's financial affairs.[16]

"Things came to a head," Meyer remembers, "when Steve got angry with me because he saw me as less than welcoming to the CEO of a for-profit hospital chain whom he had brought in to assess possible interest in buying the hospital."[14] The hospital had been profitable in the fiscal year ending June 1994.[17] "The best time to sell," observed the president.[14] Meyer felt his authority dwindling,[15] as Trachtenberg's enthusiasm for him waned.[16]

Then when Trachtenberg and Katz announced to the medical affairs committee of the board in February 1995 that the hospital would be sold, "for me, that was the end," said Meyer. "I called my attorney and said, 'Get me out of this,'"[15] and Meyer resigned after only eighteen months on the job.[17,18*] Trachtenberg, who had grown dissatisfied with what his choice for vice president was accomplishing, agreed that it was best that Meyer leave.[16] The hospital's chief executive and chief medical officers resigned soon afterwards.[14,19]

Allan Weingold remembers that the interregnum that followed Meyer's leaving was "a deadly time for the clinical faculty."[20] Many left, some going to Georgetown and others into private practice.[21] Dr. Harold Fox, whom Meyer had recruited from the Columbia University College of Physicians and Surgeons to chair the department of obstetrics and gynecology at GW, left after eighteen months to become chairman of the department at Johns Hopkins.†

Weingold, who was acting vice president before Meyer and would return to the job temporarily after he left, describes Meyer as "brilliant, but he didn't understand the relationship between his position and that of the president and board chair. Roger wanted total autonomy and independence,"[20] which Trachtenberg confirms.[22] "Roger saw himself as better than us. He was right. I thought I could handle him, but he was willful and didn't understand the reporting relationship."[22]

Meyer, according to Trachtenberg, tried to fix his problems with the president by convincing the trustees to create an independent corporation for the medical center with him as president, a project that the trustees

---

*Meyer is now the CEO of Best Practice Project Management, Inc., an opinion leadership consulting and project management company in Bethesda, Maryland.

†Although Fox's move to Baltimore is one that few academic physicians or surgeons could resist, his recruitment to GW suggests that Meyer was beginning to secure—and arguably would continue to secure had he stayed—the type of quality leadership from first-class institutions that the clinical departments had been unable to obtain in the past nor seldom would in the future.

rejected.[22] Meyer specifically refutes the president's story or that he ever tried "to run around the president to the trustees. I never tried to convince the trustees to create an independent corporation nor communicate with individual trustees against the president. The only independent pipeline to key trustees was Lou Katz, who consistently undermined my leadership of the Medical Center."[23]

Despite his problems, several of Meyer's colleagues saw his truncated tenure as just what GW needed. "Roger was smart and open. He broke down barriers and was direct with the doctors," said Keith Ghezzi, medical director of the hospital then. "The [clinical] chairs didn't want to hear what he had to say about the need for research. They didn't respond well to his call for collaboration rather than competition and his pressure on the faculty to do more of the clinical work and not depend so much on the trainees."[21]

Another Meyer fan is Dr. Laligam Sekhar, the chairman of neurosurgery from 1993 to 1999, who appreciated Meyer's being "very much pro-neurosurgery and pro-neurosciences."[24]* Sekhar wondered, however, whether Meyer's plans for the clinical enterprise would succeed in Washington. "Dr. Meyer wanted MFA to develop into a true multi-specialty clinic. Washington is a very competitive environment medically, where patients are referred to individual physicians due to their reputations, rather than to the institution, which, in the case of GW, did not have such a big name."[24]

A leading investigator, with extensive National Institutes of Health (NIH) support, considered Meyer's tenure, from the perspective of research, "eighteen golden months. Roger was our last chance to move the place up."

Medical School Administration

For the next two years the leading jobs at the medical center were filled by acting executives. Trachtenberg then appointed anesthesiologist and critical care physician John Williams Jr. as vice president. An alumnus of the medical school and its training programs, Williams had served in several positions in the vice president's and dean's offices and at the hospital.

Alan Wasserman, chairman of the department of medicine and chair-

*Sekhar is vice chairman of the department of neurological surgery at the University of Washington School of Medicine in Seattle.

man of the search that led to Williams's appointment, describes the process as proceeding "relatively quickly" in part because Trachtenberg involved himself early in the process.[25] He picked the search firm and interviewed all candidates on their first visits. The ground rules stated that either the committee or Trachtenberg could veto any candidate after the first visit. Of the eight to ten candidates interviewed initially, "we mutually agreed to veto three or four," Wasserman remembers. Of the five who remained, two withdrew to accept jobs elsewhere.

Williams then became the leading candidate. "Skip sold himself on his financial, managerial, and public health side," said Wasserman. He had "kept the clinical side running" when in acting positions and "he interviewed terrifically."[26] Trustees admired how he had helped during the process of selling the hospital, and, according to trustee Joseph Brand, "Skip earned our respect."[27]

Williams's greatest political strength was his longstanding relationship with Trachtenberg, starting at Boston University, where Williams had received his undergraduate degree and Trachtenberg, a faculty member, was his mentor. Williams was married in Trachtenberg's house.[28] As an African American, Williams was seen as particularly suitable to lead a medical center in a city with a large black population. His appointment would also help to refute the impression that GW was "a Jewish school."[29] Williams's biggest limitation for the vice president's job was his lack of experience as an investigator. The committee sent two names to the president—the inside candidate was Williams—and, despite the academic issue, Trachtenberg chose the local man.

Williams assumed the position in November 1997; he had been interim vice president since January. Williams was also dean of the medical school until 2003, when Trachtenberg named him provost to act as president in Trachtenberg's absence. Being provost, however, did not make Williams the chief academic officer of the university, a responsibility that this title includes at many universities.[26] More recently, however, Trachtenberg has considered giving Williams those duties as well.[22]*

*Some find the Williams-Trachtenberg friendship too close for the good of the medical school. Present and former GW faculty and trustees have said:
- "He's there because he's Steve's buddy."
- "What Steve wants, Skip gives him."
- "Skip is Trachtenberg's guy."

Compared with the work of the medical school dean, Williams sees him-self as "the outside guy, dealing with the politics and setting a common vision."[30] Distribution of the support that the federal government gives to the hospital for graduate medical education "flows through me," he ex-plains.[30] Williams is a member of the board of directors of Universal Health Services, Inc., which owns 80 percent of the university hospital.

In the year before Williams took over, the medical center lost more than $20 million, most of it in the old hospital[30] while MFA, the full-time physi-cians' faculty practice plan, and the HMO produced smaller losses.[31] "I was told to fix it," Williams said, "and to balance the budget in three years."[30] The hospital had been sold in 1997, so its losses no longer appeared on Williams's budget. Two years later, he closed the five suburban primary care clinics that the medical center had formed to encourage referrals to the full-time faculty and university hospital. As Williams observed, "their patients still went to the community hospitals," a feature that several academic medical center chief executives were discovering characterized the practice in suburban clinics owned by downtown institutions.[32] The clinics had lost $3 million in fiscal year 1999.[33]

Williams laid off five hundred staff members and fifty doctors and, in 2000, spun off MFA. Its losses would no longer contribute to the red ink of the medical center. He closed the money-losing HMO two years later. On operations, except in 1999 and 2000 when it still owned MFA and be-fore Williams could complete his changes, the medical center incurred small losses or surpluses, each less than $1.1 million from fiscal years 2001 to 2005.

When including one-time, non-operational expenses, however, the numbers did not look as agreeable. The total losses were significant: $38.9 million in 1999, $51.8 million in 2000, $14.6 million in 2001, and $7.4 million in 2002.[33] Since the university had agreed to help the separate MFA get started financially with bridging funds,[34] transferring the accounts re-ceivable and cash in the university-owned practice plan to the independent MFA in 2000 cost the medical center about $35 million. Closing the health plan during 2001 and 2002 cost $12.7 million.[33] With completion of such one-time expenses, the total loss decreased to $2.7 million in fiscal year 2003, $2.6 million in 2004, and $2.6 million in 2005,[33] "without the state to bail us out," as one of the basic science chairmen complained.[35] The trustees, according to the chairman Charles Manatt, "were exuberant with relief and joy" to be free of these money-draining enterprises.[34]

The medical center remains obliged to repay the university for the losses of previous years, a loan that eventually climbed to almost $120 million.[33] This obligation that the university continues to insist be repaid along with accumulated interest of 6.5 percent per year, severely limits the medical center's ability to invest in its improvement[30] and angers members of the medical faculty who respond, "Think of all the money we used to make for you."[36] If the university did not require that the medical center pay interest of about $6 million per year, half of which is deferred but still recorded as a medical center obligation, all of the losses from 2003 to 2005 would disappear, and the medical center would show a profit of approximately $3 million in each of those years.[33,37]

In addition to garnering credit for repairing the medical center's financial problems,[38] Williams is praised for running the medical center with a gentle, courteous hand. Patricia Berg, an associate professor in one of the basic science departments, says, "Skip and I know each other," unlike at the university where she previously worked, where "the dean never knew me. This is a much more friendly place.[39] The salary I received at GW was actually about $2,000 more than I had asked for. It made me feel very appreciated."[40]

Despite his accomplishments, however, Williams does not escape criticism. He is held responsible for the medical school's lack of financial and moral support when recruiting chairmen and medical investigators from leading medical schools, for failing to develop research, particularly in the clinical departments, and for his continuing the tenure of chairmen whose better days are behind them.

Williams's successor as dean of the school of medicine is Dr. James Scott, "a guy whom everybody likes"[41] but someone "in a job that will make him not a good guy."[42] An emergency medicine physician, Scott has won many "Golden Apple" awards, which are given by the students to faculty members whom they find to be particularly able teachers.[21]

Compared with many medical school deans Scott has limited responsibilities. Since MFA is no longer a university faculty group, it is independently governed and no longer led by the medical school. Scott, as the chief academic officer of the school, is a member of the board of directors of MFA and of its three-member compensation committee and supervises the distribution of funds for teaching among the clinical departments. "The dean can influence clinical faculty through appointments even though MFA does not report to him," explains Williams. "If the hospital wants to fire a faculty member, the dean and then I must agree."[30] But that is not the same as being the senior officer of the clinical departments and their members. This means that Scott, if he wished to do so, cannot effectively influence these departments and MFA to support research. Williams acknowledges that "we lost our leverage. Jim can always be outvoted."[12] Scott retains authority for academic programs in the clinical and basic science departments with their 130 scientists, although, like most of the recent leaders in both the dean's and the vice president's offices, he is primarily a clinician-educator and not an investigator.[31,41,43]

With divestiture of the hospital, the practice plan, and the HMO, each of which was formerly directed by the dean, "we have become a much smaller enterprise," he acknowledges.[44] As psychiatrist David Reiss puts it, "we have become a vestige of a medical school."[45] The school's leaders now concentrate on education and research and no longer direct the other elements of a typical academic medical center.[46]

"No Culture of Research"

Education, not research, has traditionally been the primary activity at George Washington University although, more recently, research has been growing in importance in several of its schools. "We're 150 years late in research development," says trustee Philip Amsterdam. "Why? Not enough money."[47] The same is true at the medical school, which is predominately a clinical school where research has not been emphasized as much as at the research-intensive schools.

In 2005, the NIH awarded investigators at GW's medical school $15,715,685 for 45 grants and contracts, which placed it 97th of 123 medical schools (79th percentile) in that year.[48]* The medical school's standing has changed little during the past 3 decades. For example in 1970, GW's medical school ranked 85th[49] of the 103 (81st percentile) schools operating that year.[50]† Most of the schools lower on the NIH list are state-owned; few

---

*This was less than in 2004, when the NIH awarded GW $19,204,556 for 59 grants and contracts, which placed it 92nd of 123 medical schools (75th percentile) in that year.[48]

In 2004, the basic science departments, each of which had NIH support, generated $11,020,624. They ranked (number of schools with such departments in parentheses): anatomy and cell biology—45 (90), biochemistry—84 (109), pathology—86 (98), pharmacology and physiology—69 (101). Three of the 13 clinical departments had NIH support of $4,209,101; 10 had none.[48]

†Although there are other criteria for measuring the research funding of medical schools, the

are private like George Washington. No member of George Washington's medical faculty is a member of the Institute of Medicine or the National Academy of Sciences.

"GW has traditionally been viewed as a place to get a good medical education," said one of the basic science chairmen. "It was never seen as a high-powered research institution. Still true today."[51] In president Trachtenberg's words, "we train decent physicians but are invisible in research,"[22] but, he adds, "I'm tired of the implication that creating first-rate docs, and also physicians' assistants, is something I am supposed to be embarrassed about."[52]*

This lack of research probably contributes to the limited recognition of GW among faculty at more prestigious medical schools. When Dr. Gerald Lazarus, a senior member of the faculty in dermatology at the Johns Hopkins University School of Medicine and one of the top graduates of the GW medical school class of 1963, was interviewed for an internship at one of the most competitive Eastern medical schools, the chairman of medicine asked him, "How do you like St. Louis?" confusing GW for Washington University. When Lazarus told him that the school was not in St. Louis, the chairman said, "then Seattle [University of Washington]?" Informed that GW was in Washington, D.C., the interviewer said, "Oh, I'm sorry," and then, compounded his mistakes by adding, "Your Proc Harvey is one of the greatest cardiologists around." W. Proctor Harvey was then chief of cardiology at Georgetown.[54]†

The most frequent explanations given at GW for the medical school's disappointing standing in research are:[11,28,31,33,35,36,41-44,51,54-65]

NIH's ranking is generally considered the most relevant—particularly, one should add, by those institutions that rank high. NIH grants are among the most competitive to obtain, compared with, for example, grants from industry to evaluate the effectiveness of new drugs.

*"In twenty years," Trachtenberg predicts, "GW medical school will be a recognized center of research relative to its modest starting point and its limited space in downtown Washington. We will see aggressive and robust growth, and the young School of Public Health in two decades will be a national contender. New facilities currently well along in the planning stage will be erected and will help to make the difference—also, new modes of faculty recruitment and compensation. But the school will continue to honor its commitment to teaching and education of first-rate practitioners and clinicians with the graduation of doctors you would want to have treating your mother."[53]

†Lazarus has, during a distinguished career in dermatology, been chairman of the department at the University of Pennsylvania and dean of the school of medicine at the University of California at Davis. He is currently chairman of the department of dermatology at the Johns Hopkins Bayview Medical Center and professor of dermatology at the Hopkins medical school. In the spring of 2005, Lazarus was elected a member of the board of trustees at GW. He is the only physician and the only academic currently (June 2006) on the board.[54]

- *No "state" support,* requiring the medical school leaders to charge one of the highest tuitions in the nation. The District of Columbia has neither the financial resources nor the desire to support medical schools in general* or research specifically. The university, as a not-for-profit corporation, pays the city no taxes on its increasingly valuable land, worth, according to one of the chairmen, up to $500 million per block, "so the city thinks we're just a drain."[35]

  As dean James Scott explains, "We have no city or state politicians to fight for us. We can't even get a meeting with the mayor."[44] Scott claims that the city took two-and-a-half years to complete the zoning process for the new hospital. "The city fights us all the way."[44] That many members of the city government are African American has raised the concern that part of the problem may be racial.

- *A relatively small endowment* of $175 million, generating about $8 million annually.[33]

- *A university administration* that preferred escaping from, rather than investing in, the medical enterprise. "The university just doesn't get us," said one of the basic scientists. Medical school alumnus Gerald Lazarus has the impression that "the university leadership underestimates how critical developing a leading academic medical school is to the aspirations of GW to be a top-tier university."[54]

- *No "culture of research."*[66] "Many of our leaders have never done an experiment," one of the scientists says, "so they can't imagine what research really means." Even the presence of the NIH in nearby Bethesda is blamed as a drain on top investigators in the Washington area from choosing the medical schools as places to work. One former medical center officer, however, thinks the NIH explanation is an excuse that many faculty members and administrators use to justify the school's weakness in research.[43] Even though the NIH is easily reached from the GW campus via the Metro,[45] few members of the GW faculty collaborate with investigators there.

Allan Goldstein, the much-respected veteran chairman of biochemistry and molecular biology at GW, says, "If you come here, you can do as little as

---

*Howard University receives federal funds to fulfill its special mission of training African American doctors.

you wish. No one pushes you,"[67] and as one former faculty member said, "Nobody ever asked me what I was doing."[31]

"GW is comfortable with the mantle that we train good doctors," says Gerald Lazarus. "It is only now beginning to search for distinction and identify areas of focus that can translate into greatness. It is at the very early stages of designing programs which build faculty and student opportunities for greatness, and only time will tell if the leaders can change the institution." He observed that his alma mater's research enterprise for decades was "unfocused and underfunded."[54]

When, as a medical student, Lazarus wanted a research experience, he remembers being advised to "go find a faculty member and do some research. GW just doesn't understand that the best doctors are, or have been involved in, scholarly achievement. It's a tragedy that the considerable resources of the region in basic science, health care delivery, and policies have not been exploited." Lazarus mused, "Hopefully the new school of public health will catalyze a major investment in the health policy arena, including clinical epidemiology and health services research by the university. GW boasts world-class schools of business, international affairs, and law. What an opportunity in the nation's capital to develop a world class medical program, but that requires the commitment of the university." Explaining the lack of research emphasis in the careers of many of the GW leaders, Lazarus says, "You need to have done research to build research."[54]

As for the quality of the students, Lazarus suspects that the top 10 to 20 percent of the GW classes are the equal of the best he has encountered throughout his career. "The 'fall-off' is the difference. At GW the quality of the class begins to fall off after the top 20 percent. Here at Hopkins it's after the top 70 percent."[54]

From the mid-1980s to the mid-1990s, the school recruited few basic scientists. "No money for recruiting," explains Raymond Walsh, who became chairman of the department of anatomy in 1995 after five years as acting chairman, while the school failed in several searches in other departments to recruit chairmen from outside GW.[51] This was a time when some of the basic science departments had no external funding.* In several of the basic science departments, senior faculty members who no longer perform

---

* Each of the basic science departments has NIH funding now.[48]

research carry much of the teaching of medical students, leaving the investigators with more time for their experiments.[51]

Successful Investigators

Dr. William Weglicki beat the length of Ray Walsh's term as interim chairman by seven years, functioning as interim chairman of the department of physiology for twelve years.[64]* The school did not have the resources to expand this small department and, looking for a basic scientist rather than a clinical leader—Weglicki is a cardiologist whose primary appointment is in the department of medicine—never made him permanent chairman. The department of physiology was dissolved in 2003 and merged with pharmacology.[64]†

In addition to a basic science department, the Washington Veterans Affairs Medical Center is another place where GW clinicians like Weglicki look for research opportunities. A good example is Dr. Charles Faselis, a general internist who studies how medical care works or does not work, a discipline known as outcomes research.

Faselis came to GW in 1998 to help direct the internal medicine residency training program. A popular teacher who received awards for this activity during most of the subsequent years, he was unable to conduct much research because of his administrative responsibilities and the necessity to earn money practicing. So, in 2005, he moved to the Washington VA hospital, which is located near the Washington Hospital Center and is affiliated with each of the city's medical schools. There, supported by a federal salary, he has time to do his research despite performing administrative duties and caring for his allotment of patients. "It's the last bastion of research possibilities here," he says.[68]

Finally, in 1997, recruitment was energized, and in the next five years twenty-four well-funded investigators were brought to GW, generally in the basic science departments.[28] Most of the new recruits came to GW as assis-

---

*Weglicki advised a colleague who was offered an acting position to take it because "it's great for job security!"[41] Seven faculty members who are, or have recently been, acting or interim chairmen served in that role for 4, 4, 5, 6, 9, 9, and 12 years. At the beginning of 2006, 5 departments—dermatology, neurosurgery, obstetrics and gynecology, ophthalmology, and pathology—had acting or interim chairs.

†The combined department's greatest strengths are in neurosciences and cardiology. Neurosciences is not an independent department at GW.[35]

tant or associate professors with grants of their own. The medical school could not afford to hire faculty who had just finished their training and brought no support with them.[35,69] Young investigators with their own grants are among academic medicine's most prized recruits, just the type of faculty members medical schools do not want to lose.[64] So many who decided to come to GW with its relatively weak scientific standing had reasons other than academics to move, such as the attractions of Washington or proximity to relatives.

One of the inducements GW could offer was laboratory space. The Ross building, home of the basic scientists and the medical school administration, continues to be underpopulated. "We don't know what it's like to be crowded," explains Allan Goldstein, who has chaired the department of biochemistry and molecular biology since 1978.[67]

Bill Weglicki, who has been continuously supported by the NIH and other competitive agencies, is a good example. After training at highly respected institutions, he selected GW to be closer to his children's grandparents, all of whom lived fairly nearby. The chairman of the department of medicine created for him the position of director of experimental medicine and gave him three thousand square feet of laboratory space,[64] which was available because of the freeze on basic science recruiting. Within two years, he had obtained a program project grant from the NIH that provided substantial support for faculty in the clinical and basic science departments.[70] Medical residents who wanted to do animal research found their way to Weglicki, who helped them locate a suitable facility in his or another basic science department since few members of the department of medicine performed laboratory research.[71]

In contrast to the growing research activities in the basic science departments, this leg of the traditional three-legged stool in the medical school—teaching, clinical care, and research—has never been vigorous in most of the clinical departments. Dr. Frederick Rickles, a hematologist who was associate vice president for health research, compliance, and technology transfer from 1998 to 2003, said that "without a research culture, the departments didn't recruit or appoint leaders who could develop research. Besides there was no mentoring."[28] The school offered to fund some investigators in the clinical departments if the practice plan would match the money. Medical Faculty Associates refused. "It was a self-fulfilling prophecy," Rickles said.[28]

When Rickles left GW to become executive director of the Federation of American Societies for Experimental Biology (FASEB) in Bethesda, he was succeeded, after the usual interregnum, by Anne Hirshfield, then the assistant dean for research at the University of Maryland School of Medicine. Despite the relatively primitive state of research at GW, at least by comparison with what she was familiar at Maryland, she found "the people so nice and considerate to each other. They're friendly, no prima donnas."[57] Others agree that GW is a particularly informal place. "I'm on a first-name basis with everyone," says one investigator."[45]

Soon after arriving, however, Hirshfield discovered significant shortcomings in the school's communication network. "No information about what people are doing. The e-mail doesn't work that well, and the IRB [the institutional review board that evaluates the soundness and ethics of research proposals] is completely paper-based [rather than computerized]."[57]

Chairmen and others complain about the inefficiency of the research administration, which Hirshfield has been charged to improve. "It's hard to get money out of the university for industrial contracts, particularly," complains John Kelly, chairman of the department of neurology. "It can take six to twelve months. At least that's an improvement. I remember when two to three years was common. Red tape and redundant paperwork are major problems at this university."[72]

Separation of the hospital and the practice plan from the university has increased the number of organizations that must approve applications to perform clinical research from one (the medical school) to three (medical school, hospital, and practice plan).[69] When other hospitals participate, their approval must also be obtained. As one of the chairmen said, "In the old days, we just had to go to the dean. Now there are many more people who must sign off." Remembering the efficient leadership of one official, the dean/CEO, at Hopkins[73] from where he was recruited to GW as chairman of urology, Thomas Jarrett observed, "At GW there are three leaders with equal authority."[74] One of the senior clinicians who left for another job said, "It's not an organization. It's a disorganization, a three-headed monster. It's rare when the three parts concur about anything."[75]*

---

* "The administrative hassles are severe and have led to the balkanization of the medical center," says a current member of the faculty. "The worst result of this is how it reduces the likelihood of attracting major academic stars to chair the clinical departments since under the new arrangement they may gain partial control of Bosnia but Herzegovina, Serbia, Montenegro, and Kosovo are lost forever."

As John Kelly, the chairman of neurology, puts it, "This problem is symptomatic of the larger problem at GW, where you play a game of roulette with the entities. They simply keep passing the buck around the circle until you give up. No one at the administrative level has been willing to take the leadership to solve these problems."[72]

Dr. David Reiss, the psychiatrist with more NIH grants than anyone in the clinical departments, did not transfer to MFA but kept his primary appointment in the school of medicine.* As with many of the other successful investigators at GW, Reiss is there for personal as much as for professional reasons. "Several of us at the NIH were homeless," Reiss remembers, and needed another place to work, preferably nearby. "Our kids were happy in the Montgomery [County] schools." So in 1974, Reiss moved to GW as professor in the department of psychiatry and behavioral sciences and two years later became the director of its division of research. He continued to develop the studies he had started at the NIH in environmental and genetic influences on development and psychosocial aspects of chronic physical illness and disability, among other subjects. Reiss also completed his training in psychoanalysis and continues to practice this specialty. Although offered the chairmanship at other medical schools, Reiss has always refused. "I'm an old researcher, couldn't do both."[45]

Despite spending most of his career at GW, Reiss has had to tolerate several administrative problems, for example:[45]

- *Tenure and appointments.* Though awarding tenure to his colleagues, the university has, until recently, wavered on its pledge to pay 30 percent of their salaries and provide "bridging" support for those who lost their grants. New faculty appointments to his division, to replace outgoing faculty, have been almost impossible to obtain and, once obtained, are not backed up with sufficient funds.
- *His salary.* When Reiss turned down an attractive job as department chair at an Ivy League medical school, Trachtenberg arranged to have his salary supported by university rather than grant funds. However, this commitment was not fully honored in recent years

---

*Few faculty members have had similar educational experiences and professional accomplishments before joining GW—B.A., Harvard, summa cum laude, Phi Beta Kappa; M.D., Harvard, summa cum laude for thesis in a special field; psychiatry training at the Massachusetts Mental Health Center, Boston, a Harvard affiliate; trainee and staff member at the National Institute of Mental Health; teaching analyst of the Washington Psychoanalytic Institute.

until "a recent, prolonged and exhausting protest by me and our departmental chair" led to its realization.[76] Receiving university support for his salary would allow Reiss to direct more financial assistance to his research and to his faculty and staff.[76]

- *Space.* Reiss's laboratory, he reports, "was moved from the main research building to an ancillary building after prolonged planning to move it to the new hospital and threats to move it to an office building at a great distance from the campus."[76]

- *Culture.* "Obtaining resources to conduct research at GW comes grudgingly and slowly. Much pushing is required," Reiss says. "It's very frustrating." The reasons, he believes, are "the absence of a culture of research and the lack of a research background in the university's and medical school's leadership."[43]

Another distinguished scientist, who, unlike Reiss, who has spent much of his career after training at GW, is Dr. Peter Hotez,* who was recruited from Yale in 2000 to lead the department of microbiology and tropical medicine. Hotez moved because he wanted to work in Washington, a decision encouraged by the Gates Foundation, which supports much of his work. GW found Hotez a particularly attractive addition to the faculty because, in addition to his distinction as a medical scientist, Hotez was fully funded and would cost the medical school relatively little money. Laboratory and office space, vacated by departing faculty who had not been replaced, was available.[59]† Hotez believes that the medical school should "take advantage of where we are and focus on a few areas like global health, genomics, and health policy. We're in the center of world health." The deans of both the medical and public health schools agree.[38,44]

Hotez explains that the memory of the financial turmoil of the 1990s accounts for the risk-adverse character of the university and the medical school. "Now that things have stabilized, the administration doesn't want to take the chance that we might slip back to where we were then."[59] The

---

*B.A., Yale, Ph.D., Rockefeller, M.D., Cornell, clinical training in pediatrics at the Massachusetts General Hospital.

†Hotez and his group have become one of the most productive research departments at the medical school. As he reports, "Our Human Hookworm Vaccine Initiative has been very successful at GWU, publishing sixty peer-reviewed papers since my coming here in 2000. We have now successfully filed an IND [Investigational New Drug] application with the FDA [Food and Drug Administration] and have developed a first-generation hookworm vaccine that has gone through clinical trials. Very few academic centers can boast this."[77]

same former clinical chairmen and recruitees, who criticized certain fea-tures of the independent MFA (see above), also expressed reservations about GW's research programs.

- "I saw an accelerating disincentive among the clinical faculty to do any academics."
- "I wondered if my energy to do research would be drained off by all the troubles at GW."
- Regarding the recruitment of chairmen and faculty members from research institutions, MFA "would blow them off, and they wouldn't come. They were here to do clinical work, not research. MFA would give new recruits only six to twelve months of support until they were on their own, significantly less than research-intensive medical schools guarantee."

Children's National Medical Center

The most successful research enterprise within George Washington med-icine is at the Children's National Medical Center. The connection, how-ever, is more academic than organizational. Children's is an independent not-for-profit corporation affiliated with, but not owned by, GW. The fac-ulty there constitute GW's pediatrics department, have GW professorial appointments, and train the GW students. The 325 members of the Chil-dren's faculty comprise about half of all the full-time faculty in the medical school. Unlike the now independent MFA at GW, the practice plan at Chil-dren's remains within the hospital.

Research is administered separately from the university. The hospital's, not the university's, institutional review board (IRB) evaluates the research performed at Children's, which submits grant applications directly to the NIH and other agencies. The pediatrics department at Children's receives more money from the NIH than all the other departments of the medical school combined, according to Dr. Mark Batshaw, the chairman.[55]* Because

---

*Batshaw reports that during 2004, his hospital ranked fifteenth in NIH grants among all de-partments of pediatrics, including independent children's hospitals, and seventh among indepen-dent children's hospitals.[55] Since the NIH lists Children's grants among independent and children's hospitals rather than medical schools, GW's ranking does not benefit from the amount of funding that the NIH awards to Children's. If it did, and the total NIH funding during fiscal 2004 at Children's of $17,140,802[78] were added to GW's $19,204,556,[48] the ranking of GW would rise from 92 to 77.

of the faculty's success in obtaining grants and the hospital's solid financial status, the pediatrics service for GW costs the university nothing.[55]

Washington's children's hospital was founded in 1872—only Boston Children's and Children's Hospital of Philadelphia are older—and was first located in downtown Washington at Fourteenth and F streets.[79] In the 1970s the Washington Hospital Center invited Children's to move to its campus two miles north of the Capitol to bring a pediatrics service there. Children's first hospital building in the new location opened in 1977. Children's now has 270 beds, 4,000 employees, and an annual budget of $500 million. Each year it admits 11,000 patients and cares for 400,000 outpatients. "We provide 80 percent of the medical services for the district's children," Batshaw says.[55]

Children's in Washington has managed to organize its services along programmatic in addition to departmental and divisional lines, a scheme that other academic medical centers have tried to institute with difficulty. There are six "Centers of Excellence" each with its own director: community pediatric health; hospital-based specialties; neuroscience and behavioral medicine; surgical care; heart, lung, and kidney disease; and cancer and blood disorders. Within each center are the usual subspecialty divisions, led by the appropriate specialist. Batshaw is the academic chairman of all the centers and divisions, including the surgical specialties despite his being a medical pediatrician. The research is administered in the Children's Research Institute, which Batshaw, who as the chief academic officer of the hospital, also directs.[55]*

Education

The medical school faculty have long prided themselves on the quality of the teaching.[21,43] "The students are excellent clinically since they're learning from real doctors," said a former member of the faculty.[11] "We have a very

---

*Unlike many of GW's medical faculty, Batshaw came to Children's from highly competitive academic medical centers, including Johns Hopkins and Children's Hospital of Philadelphia, which, like Children's of Washington, is a corporation separate from its academic affiliate, the University of Pennsylvania.[80] When it became time for him to be a department chairman, Batshaw chose Washington Children's because "I saw the place as a sleeping giant. Unlike in the Philadelphia area, there's only one children's hospital in and around Washington, and its finances were solid." Batshaw moved because of the opportunities Children's offered, not because of the academics at GW.[55]

diverse student body, which makes them less competitive with each other. Diversity creates more interests," said one of the current chairmen.[35]

Education is, and seems to have been throughout its history, the principal emphasis of GW's medical school. University president Stephen Trachtenberg has been heard to say, "Education should be our role. Research is not one of our primary interests."[67]

The new hospital, with its own educational component in addition to new inpatient facilities, helps GW attract more competitive students and trainees.[41,81] The medical school owns most of the top, sixth floor except for a small psychiatric unit run by the hospital.[20] The floor contains a standardized patient examining room, a surgical simulation room, and several conference rooms to which patients may be brought for the instruction of students and trainees.[44]

Leaders of the department of medicine believe that the new hospital,[81] and GW's location in Washington,[68] appeal to potential interns and residents. In addition, training at the Fairfax Hospital—a successful community hospital in Northern Virginia—the Washington Veterans Affairs Medical Center and the clinical services at the NIH provide opportunities that students and trainees appreciate. Dr. Jehan (Gigi) El-Bayoumi, who directs the program, explains: "We have a diverse house staff in under-represented minorities—single, married with kids, and those holding Ph.D., M.D., and J.D.-M.D. degrees. And we're gay friendly."[81]* Although the students matched to become interns in the department of medicine tend to come from schools which, like GW, emphasize education and clinical care more than research, "our matches are better today than they were six years ago," according to MFA CEO Stephen Badger.†

There are those who question the effects of this emphasis on medical education. "What's the proof that we train students better than other places?" asks one of the chairmen. He wonders whether the importance of education is used as a justification for a lack of success in research. Despite

---

*GW is a "comfortable place for someone like me who's gay and openly so," says Jeffrey Akman, the chairman of psychiatry. "It's a total non-issue. We're the hospital for Dupont Circle [where many gays live] and have always had many gays with AIDS among our patients."[41] Akman praises executive vice president John Williams for his attitude on this issue and for the medical school's sponsorship of gay and lesbian meetings. "Skip's great about this," Akman says.[41]

†In the group that became medical interns in 2005, 27 percent received their medical degrees from GW.[81]

the prominence that the school claims it places on clinical education, there is little supervision of the teaching, according to another chairman.[56]

University Administration

Since August 1, 1988, the president of George Washington University has been Stephen Joel Trachtenberg.[82]* Born in Brooklyn, Trachtenberg attended the local public schools, Columbia (B.A., 1959, Phi Beta Kappa), Yale (J.D., 1962), and Harvard (master's in public administration, 1966). After several years of service with the federal government, he spent eight years at Boston University (BU), where he worked for the controversial BU president John Silber and became vice president for academic services and academic dean of the college of liberal arts. Trachtenberg was then president of Hartford University for eleven years† before becoming the fifteenth president of GW. Throughout his career, Trachtenberg has emphasized academic administration rather than research.‡

Trachtenberg receives both praise and criticism, as might be expected of someone in his position. [7,13,14,26-28,31,35,36,38,42,59,63,85-101] All agree that he is very smart and charming, "a remarkable man," and, as one trustee said, he "brought a new sense of energy" to GW. Other trustees say that "he's fantastic, has made the university much more prominent," "he's always coming up with new ideas," and describe him as being "terrific at outreach." A close associate observed, "Steve lives his job and worries about GW all the time."

The president, his associates say, knows what he wants but "doesn't bother you if you're doing your job," "may not tell you what you want to hear, but does it forthrightly," and "never shrinks from a complex problem." One of the trustees added, "Steve doesn't meddle, a good rule for a president."

An excellent speaker, Trachtenberg is seen as colorful, enthusiastic, and flamboyant, "a character, with a great sense of humor," "a mensch" and

---

*In April 2006, Trachtenberg announced that he would resign the presidency effective in the summer of 2007. Having served by then as the GW president for twenty years, Trachtenberg will become president emeritus and a professor in the school of public policy and public administration.[83]

†In having been president at two institutions, Trachtenberg was participating in an historical tradition at GW. Cloyd Heck Marvin, GW's longest-serving president (1927–59), had been president of the University of Arizona. Lloyd Hartman Elliott, previously president of the University of Maine, led GW from 1965 until Trachtenberg took over in 1988.

‡For further details about Trachtenberg's career, see note 84.

even "a frustrated Borscht Belt comedian." A visitor from another medical center said, "You can't help but like him."

Seen as a "dominant personality" and someone "who means what he says," Trachtenberg, perhaps accordingly, appears to some as pompous and arrogant, that he "has an ego as big as Washington," "doesn't listen," "talking with him is like talking to a real estate developer," "is too autonomous making decisions," and "is often wrong, never in doubt." His fans, however, describe the rough edges of his personality with affection and respect:

- "He's like a kid in a candy store."
- "Steve sees opportunities everywhere, in the newspapers and from people he meets. The more challenging the conundrum, the more ingenious the solution."
- "He likes lots of things going on at the same time."
- "Steve can be like a target. 'Shoot me right here,' he says and points to the center of his forehead."
- "He wants to be thought of as the toughest kid on the block, but he's really not."

In Trachtenberg, GW had selected a very different kind of leader. His predecessor, Lloyd Elliott, had grown up in Appalachia, where his father was a rural school teacher. Elliott received his undergraduate degree at Glenville State College in central West Virginia, where, as he remembers, the tuition was $25 per semester. He took a master's degree at West Virginia University and a doctorate in education at the University of Colorado. Before coming to GW in 1965, he had been a member of the faculty at Cornell University and then president of the University of Maine.[102] Trustees who had served under both Elliott and his successor said of him:[27,86,89]

- "A very courtly type of gentleman."
- "A lovely man."
- "Elliott governed GW carefully. The place was quiet, essentially a night school."
- "The conservative guy from West Virginia had been succeeded by the kid from Brooklyn."

One of Trachtenberg's first actions when he arrived was to double the traditionally low tuition, not a particularly popular decision.[85] He used many of the new funds to invest in the undergraduate experience, by building dormitories and improving the arts and sciences faculty. By enhancing facilities for students living on campus, he enabled the university to decrease the numbers of commuters, thereby converting Columbian College —the original name of the university now preserved for the undergraduate division—into a predominately residential college.* He has also phased out some of the master's degree programs for which the students had traditionally met in the afternoons, often because the university has no classrooms available for them during the rest of the day.† Along with these improvements, some of the faculty believe that he has neglected graduate studies and research as a whole while emphasizing the undergraduate part of his job. "The deans he hires are not researchers," observed one of them.

Few deny that Trachtenberg has been an excellent president for the university as a whole. In the opinion of his former boss, John Silber of Boston University, "Steve has largely transformed GW from a sleepy, commuter school. He's improved faculty recruitment and consolidated finances."[103] Donna Shalala, president of the University of Miami and secretary of the department of Health and Human Services during both Clinton administrations, acknowledges that "I'm a fan. It takes a big man to do all he's done. He's leading a big urban institution of increasingly good quality."[100] Trachtenberg believes that he has "changed the whole sociology of GW. No more pulling of the forelock."[22]

Although Trachtenberg trained and worked at universities with academic medical centers—his responsibilities at Boston University, however, did not include the medical school or hospital there[103]—and was a trustee of the Hartford Hospital, his priorities, shared with many members of his board, do not include medicine.[94] They do include the George Washington University Law School, to which the lawyer-president has paid particular attention, leading one former medical school chairman to challenge him: "You know what a first-class law school is. Why not a first-class medical school?"[104]

Soon after arriving at GW, Trachtenberg, not alone among university presidents, made it clear that he believed that the medical side of the univer-

---

*George Washington University has approximately 23,500 students—9,500 undergraduates and 14,000 graduate students. About 36 percent of the undergraduates who apply are admitted, and of these about one-third matriculate.[66]

†Most classes at the school of public health start at 3:00 p.m. for the same reason.[38]

sity had too much power and that he was going to do something about it. The president's attitude about his medical enterprise was well demonstrated by his noting that Princeton, despite its excellence as a university, has no medical school[31] and that Harvard does not own any teaching hospitals.[41,95]

Trachtenberg's objections were based on the practical consideration that GW's medical center was losing money.* The trustees, he said, "had been generous watching the losses there."[22] Finally, unwilling to continue supporting the red ink at the university hospital, the clinical faculty's practice plan, and the HMO, the trustees, according to Trachtenberg, "instructed me to kill them."[22] The president proceeded to see to it that they were sold or, in the case of the HMO, closed, leaving only the medical school within the university's purview.†

Referring to the role of the trustees in these divestments, Trachtenberg has written, "One needs the discipline of an outside organization like a board to get things done. Everybody needs a super-ego." Up until then, he believes that many at GW were indulging in "denial and magical thinking. If we wait, it'll fix itself. Being in health-care delivery, or 'clinical commerce,' was going to send the rest of the university to the poorhouse. It was a life or death situation."[105] The sales, also in Trachtenberg's words, "liberate[d] us from the former distractions of competing with for-profit hospitals, huge health plans like Aetna and the Blues, and private imaging centers run by businessmen, among others. . . . Survival is truly my topic."[105]

Trachtenberg, remembering when many university hospitals were "cash cows,"[36] wanted GW's hospital and practice plan "to make money for the university," an unlikely scenario as financial pressures assailed all hospitals and doctors' practices by the 1990s. The health plan was also expected to support the university despite the plan's goal of paying as little as possible to providers, which included GW's hospital and doctors.

When one clinical chairman criticized the shortcomings of the medical center, Trachtenberg, whom many in the medical school distrust, said, "What are you complaining about? I built you a new hospital, didn't I?"[22]

---

*When approached by Dr. Mark Hochberg, a cardiac surgeon from New Jersey who wanted to switch careers and learn the university president trade, Trachtenberg replied, "I'll teach you how to be a president if you'll explain to me why my vice president just informed me that the medical center lost $26 million."[92]

†The university had previously closed its schools of nursing and pharmacy.

Comments like this fueled the criticism of many of his medical school colleagues that their president does not care very much about what happens where they work.

The Board of Trustees; Philanthropy

Trachtenberg likes to say that he was responding to pressure from the trustees to sell the hospital, close the HMO, and separate from the practice plan. Some, though not all, of the trustees with whom I spoke, however, said that the impetus to do these things came primarily from Trachtenberg and his executive vice president Louis Katz, not from the board. Some suggest that he kept the trustees inadequately informed about the process. "Though it has been a success story," said one, "the process was flawed."

Trachtenberg's relationship with his board brings out interesting comments from the trustees, some of whom believe he "resents his board," for he has been heard to say, "I don't want a board." The president's modus operandi, according to one of the trustees, can be stated as "How can I use them to accomplish what I need?"

Part of Trachtenberg's frustration with the board, which he shares with former president Lloyd Elliott, was the trustees' unwillingness, until fairly recently, to engage in much fundraising, a problem that over the years has helped to account for GW's small endowment. Elliott remembers that, on becoming president in 1965, he inherited only $8 million.[102] Elliott's predecessor, who had been president for thirty-two years from 1927 to 1959, did little fundraising and believed that the university should depend financially on the tuition it charged, a dependence that continues, at least partially, to this day.[102] The trustees did not actively participate in raising for, or contributing money to, the university. One of them, the president of the district's largest bank and so well known that he was called "Mr. Washington," never made a single financial contribution during his eighteen years as a trustee.[102] The trustees "just went from dinner to dinner every three months," Elliott said.[102] "When I joined the board soon after Steve took over," said one of the trustees, "some of them seldom came to the meetings."[90]* When Elliott pushed the trustees to personally contribute

---

*Another trustee remembers, however, that Elliott "wanted a rubber-stamp board and was much more formal with us than Steve. He certainly didn't entertain the board like Steve does."[89]

and solicit donations, "I was seen as a money grabber."[102] Despite these difficulties, Elliott pressed on, and by the time his successor arrived in 1988, the endowment had grown to $200 million.[102] By 2005, it was $823 million.[106]*

The university presidents are not the only ones who have had problems with the trustees. At the medical center the board has more than its share of detractors. "It's made up of lawyers and business types, few if any doctors,"† according to Skip Williams, the provost and vice president for health affairs. Others at the medical center find board chairman Charles Manatt to be "autocratic and difficult." He is said to have a troubled relationship with Trachtenberg. Until the board adopted term limits recently—which do not apply to several "grandfathered" trustees[96]—Manatt had been a trustee for more than twenty-five years[34] and Patricia Gurne since 1982.[89]

It is the general opinion in the medical school that most members of the board contribute little of their own money to the university and avoid fundraising, a shortcoming also attributed to the president.[26,93]‡ One of the chairmen added, "There are no high-level types on the board.§ They're very disengaged. There's a wall between them and us."[59]

"The trustees see asking for money somehow distasteful," believes medical school dean James Scott. "Steve has a hard time saying 'we need your help.'"[44] Despite what some of his critics at the medical school claim, Trachtenberg consistently tries to raise money.[16] "Steve doesn't like to be

---

*In 2005, George Washington's endowment ranked sixty-ninth among the nation's college and universities.[106]

†Radiation oncologist Luther Brady (B.A., 1946; M.D., 1948) served as the alumni member from 1997 until he became an emeritus trustee in 2003, and Dr. Gerald Lazarus (M.D. class of 1963) became a trustee in 2005. Previously, there was usually one physician, often an alumnus of the medical school, on the board and on the committee for the medical center.[107]

‡Laurel Price Jones, the vice president for advancement at George Washington, provided the following information about contributions by trustees and the work of the president, which counters the impressions of critics in the medical school: "Trustee giving over the past 10 years amounts to approximately $25 million. Within the past few years, there have been two gifts from trustees at the $5 million level, several at the $2 and $3 million level and many at the $1 million level. Gifts like this are not received without the involvement of the president.[108]

"President Trachtenberg has been responsible for an increase in giving over the past 18 years that is remarkable: from total receipts of less than $20 million in 1988 to attainment of more than $67 million in the year ending June 30, 2006. He has never refused an opportunity to raise money for GW and, believe me, he is not shy about asking. In addition, he makes his own gifts, thereby setting a wonderful example. As a result of work he has done over the past nearly two decades, we have a great story to tell and the opportunity to raise even more in the future."[109]

§Price Jones also disagrees with this impression. "There are many 'high-level types' by any definition."[108]

rejected," trustee Nelson Carbonell explains. "None of us do, but that's a part of fundraising."[05]

Trachtenberg agrees with many of these criticisms. "We don't bring in enough money. We haven't enough wealthy alumni who can give big dollars, and there's no corporate base here. Washington's not the home of entrepreneurs."[22] Although, in the past, the members of the board were not in the habit of regularly donating to the university, "now" according to one of the longtime trustees, "100 percent of the board contributes each year."[96] Grateful patients treated at the university hospital have seldom been solicited to donate money for the medical school or for the hospital when it was owned by the university.[107]

Carbonell, the CEO of a "mezzanine lender" that raises money for small and medium-size businesses, recently joined the board and is now chairman of the development committee. The oldest of seven siblings, Carbonell, his family having limited financial resources, accepted a full scholarship to attend the engineering school at GW. Now responsible for the university's fundraising, he is working with an endowment that provides about $40,000 per student. "This is inadequate compared with that of the universities with which GW compares itself," he admits. "Because our debt just about equals our endowment, the university has little cash."[85] Half of the endowment is invested in real estate that the university owns.*

One of the reasons GW has had difficulty raising money in the past is because "for a long time, most of our students were commuters, many studying for graduate degrees," says Carbonell. "The place just didn't have that full-time feeling. There was little loyalty to the place. Urban universities struggle with this."[85] Myron Curzon, another trustee, agrees. "You'd be on campus for three or four hours a day and not on weekends. They didn't live it."[90] Trustee Robert Perry, who attended GW in the 1960s, remembers, "it was a community university with more night than day students."[96]

Now that is changing as GW's residential character has increased. "We just haven't had a culture of asking for money," Carbonell acknowledges. "I'm trying to change that."[85] GW has traditionally had difficulty raising large gifts. Carbonell explains: "We don't generate big donors from our professional schools."† Many of these graduates are preparing for careers

---

*GW is the largest private landowner in the district and the third overall after the federal and city governments.[85]

†Despite this, however, the medical school has been able to create five endowed chairs in the last seven years.[12]

in government, and "few can make large gifts." Nevertheless, Carbonell is optimistic. "We must challenge the trustees to give more—giving begins at home—and raise more. People give money to people more than to institutions."[85]

Stephen Trachtenberg's Successor

On December 5, 2006, George Washington University announced the election of Steven Knapp, provost and senior vice president for academic affairs at Johns Hopkins University, as GW's sixteenth president effective August 1, 2007. Knapp received his undergraduate degree at Yale University and his Ph.D. in English at Cornell University. His specialty is the literature of the English Romantic period of the late eighteenth and early nineteenth centuries. For sixteen years Knapp taught at the University of California–Berkeley before coming to Hopkins in 1994 as dean of the School of Arts and Sciences. He became provost two years later.[110,111]

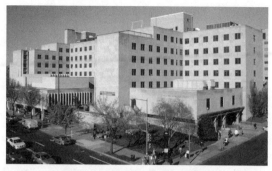

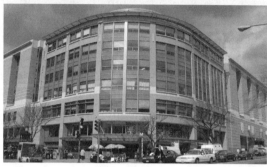

George Washington's former university hospital (*top*), which first received patients in 1948, and the new hospital (*bottom*) that Universal Health Services, Inc., built on a parking lot adjacent to the old hospital and opened in 2002. *Courtesy of George Washington University*

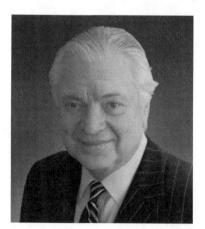 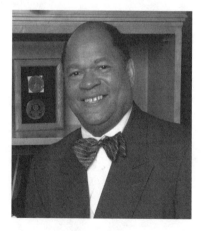

Alan Miller (*left*), founder and CEO of the company that bought the George Washington University Hospital in 1997. Dr. John ("Skip") Williams (*right*), provost and vice president for health affairs at George Washington and a member of the board of directors of Universal. *Photo of Alan Miller courtesy of Universal Health Services, Inc.; photo of John Williams courtesy of George Washington University*

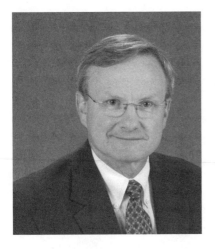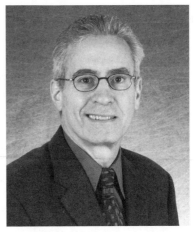

Dr. James Scott (*left*), dean of the George Washington University School of Medicine, whose responsibilities do not include the University Hospital or Medical Faculty Associates (MFA), the practice plan for the full-time faculty. Dr. Alan Wasserman (*right*), the cardiologist who is chairman of the independent MFA and the Department of Medicine. *Courtesy of George Washington University*

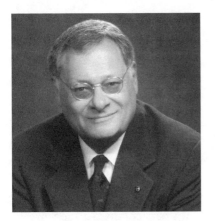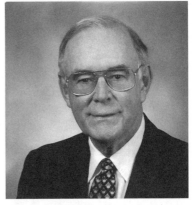

When George Washington University decided to sell its university hospital and separate from its faculty practice plan, Stephen Joel Trachtenberg (*left*) was president and Charles T. Manatt (*right*) was chairman of the board of trustees. *Courtesy of George Washington University*

CHAPTER SIX

Georgetown University

Selling the Hospital

As at George Washington University, financial troubles forced Georgetown University to sell its hospital. Despite being relatively small for a university hospital,* the Georgetown University Hospital had provided reliable surpluses to the university to help support its departments and schools through the 1980s and early 1990s. In fiscal year 1995, however, the medical center lost $2.9 million, its first negative margin. Because this represented only a small fraction of the center's annual expense budget of about $500 million that year, "the board was not particularly alarmed," remembered Dr. John Griffith, executive vice president for health sciences and director of the medical center from 1986 to 1996 and executive dean from 1989 to 1996.[1] The $2.9 million was only the beginning, however. From 1995 to 2000, the medical center would lose $257 million, with the largest annual loss being $83.1 million in 1999.[2-5]†

---

*The hospital operated about three hundred beds at the time.

†The medical center's operating budget of between $500 and $600 million accounted for about two-thirds of the expenses of the university.[6]

By 1998, the university realized that it could not, by itself, conquer the problem and, after advising its academic community about the extent of the trouble, concluded that, like George Washington, it would have to look outside itself for a solution.[5]

Governance of the Medical Center

As at other universities with medical enterprises, a group of the directors, constituting the committee on medical center affairs (COMCA), governed the medical center at Georgetown. COMCA reported to the full university board.[7] The members of both the Georgetown board and the committee came from the university's national constituency. Few of the committee members lived in the Washington area.

Until the structure was changed in 1989, the governance at Georgetown was characteristic of many medical centers in which the university owned the hospital. The most senior official carried the title of "executive vice president" and for a time "chancellor." He was responsible for the hospital and the medical, dental, and nursing schools—each of which had a dean— and represented the medical center to COMCA and the president.

Milton Corn, the dean from 1985 to 1989, led the school of medicine with the same rank as the hospital director, "primus inter pares," as Corn describes the dean's status at the time. The dean and the hospital director reported to the executive vice president whose authority, however, was so limited that one observer described the job as "largely a check-off post"[8] and another as "without visible power."[9]

Corn suspects that John Griffith, when he accepted the executive vice presidency in 1986, did not fully understand that he would not directly control the school, that the university president at the time had not adequately described the structure when he hired him. Griffith came to feel that this indirect authority prevented him from fully realizing his ambitions for the medical center.[10] "He was a courteous man," Corn recalls, "but appalled that he didn't control what I controlled."[10]* With the closure of the dental school in the early years of his administration, Griffith felt

---

*Corn remembers inviting Griffith to serve on important search committees "as a courtesy. He would attend for a while, but then leave, thinking that he should be running them."[10]

that he had little to do.[11] The hospital was being led by Charles ("Chuck") O'Brien[11,12] and the medical school by Corn, a veteran and respected[11] Georgetown hematologist.*

Accordingly, in 1989, with the support of the university president Father Timothy Healy, Griffith assumed the additional title of executive dean and consolidated the powers of the dean of the medical school in his office.[10,13] The executive vice president and his staff now directed all academic, financial, and administrative operations throughout the medical center. Under the new structure, the departmental chairmen, some of whom had dominated decision making in the medical school previously,[13] now reported to the executive dean.

Griffith distributed some of the dean's traditional responsibilities among members of the faculty: for academic affairs (education), Dr. William Maxted, a urologist; for research and graduate education (training for the Ph.D. degree), Dr. Alan Faden, a neuroscientist;[7] and for clinical practice, Dr. Sam Wiesel, chairman of orthopedic surgery.[7,10]

Griffith was now ready to announce his plan, an ambitious effort to create a world-class Catholic medical research institution at Georgetown.[6,8,9,14-17] Griffith, a pediatric neurologist, wanted to bring to Georgetown the academic flavor and accomplishments that he had known at the institutions where he had trained.[18] Georgetown should emphasize research and teaching, and the hospital should help to serve these missions. To improve clinical care, a new wing would be added to the hospital. To increase research productivity, Griffith would recruit investigators,† and a new laboratory research building would be constructed.[1] Surpluses from the hospital, overheads from grants, and support from a for-profit pharmaceutical company that would occupy half of the new building would help pay for the new laboratories and faculty. Although these assumptions would eventually prove unsound, the university endorsed Griffith's plan.[8]

Described as a "lovely," "thoughtful" man, "somewhat shy and retiring," "committed to the academic enterprise,"[7] Griffith was unable to resolve the

---

*Corn, a refugee from Nazi Germany, arrived in the United States at age six speaking no English. He received his undergraduate degree with highest honors, Phi Beta Kappa in his junior year, and his M.D. degree summa cum laude, Alpha Omega Alpha also in his junior year both from Yale. Corn then trained in medicine and hematology at the Peter Bent Brigham and Johns Hopkins hospitals. He was a member of the faculty at George Washington University based at the District of Columbia General Hospital before joining Georgetown as professor of medicine in 1973.

†During his ten-year tenure, Griffith would appoint seventeen chairmen and institute directors.

challenges caused by the severe financial problems that would engulf the medical center later during his tenure.[12,15,19] As one former chairman put it, "Griffith and his associates never could correlate John's vision with Georgetown's resources."[18]

With Griffith having assumed direct responsibility for the school,[19] Milton Corn, concluding that his role had become superfluous[20]—"not the job I had taken"[10]—resigned from Georgetown in 1989.* O'Brien would resign as CEO of the hospital three years later, stimulated in part, it was said, by his perception that the university was "continually raiding the hospital's resources."[22]†

The University versus the Medical Center

"In the past, there was plenty of money to go around, enough for the humanities as well as the medical center," said Kenneth Bloem, CEO of the medical center (1996–99) after Griffith left.[24] "But when the dollars stopped flowing," according to Bloem, "the university had even less interest in the contributions of the medical center."[22]

Georgetown University has favored teaching and research in arts and sciences, law, politics, and ethics more than in medicine.[17,22] Father Healy, the president of Georgetown University from 1977 to 1989, wanted to use hospital reserves to help build dormitories and improve departments in Georgetown College, the university's school of arts and sciences.

Despite his enthusiasm for what John Griffith wanted to accomplish, Healy was seen by many in the medical school as not a particularly strong advocate of medicine at Georgetown.[25] Rather than encouraging its academic improvement, Healy was primarily concerned about retaining the medical center's Catholic character.[10] Like many university presidents, few of whom are doctors, Healy saw his medical enterprise as "a bit of a mystery," said Dr. Edmund Pellegrino, an experienced academic leader and medical ethicist who has been a Georgetown director and longtime member of the faculty. "The cultures are very different."[25]‡

---

*Corn joined the National Library of Medicine of the NIH, where he is now associate director of Extramural Programs.[21]

†On leaving Georgetown in 1992, O'Brien became president and CEO of the West Penn Hospital in Pittsburgh, around which he developed the West Penn Allegheny Health System with six hospitals, two research foundations, a large regional primary care network, 450 faculty physicians, 455 house staff, and 2 major medical school affiliations.[23]

‡Healy was an authority on John Donne and taught the students Elizabethan poetry.[12]

Many of the university's leaders, particularly in Healy's day and probably previously, considered the medical school "a trade school, not an academic endeavor,"[9,12,23,25-29] staffed by doctors "making too much money."[12] One of the senior faculty remembers Healy "telling the medical faculty that they were 'artisans and technicians,' and he did not regard building up the medical center as a high priority."[30] In the midst of the turmoil of the last half of the 1990s, Ken Bloem wondered if "Georgetown is one of those universities that shouldn't have gotten involved in medicine."[22]

The university had, over the years, shifted money from the medical center to the central university through the mechanism of university transfer charges. Despite the falling margins in the medical center, the university continued to move money from the hospital's accumulated surplus[8] to its general funds. "They [the central university administration] would simply debit the ledger of the medical center," as Bloem described the process.[22]

That the dean's tax and money from the hospital supported the university is widely accepted among the medical faculty and administration to be true.[8,31-33] One of the basic scientists expresses, in his case quite scathingly, an opinion shared by many in the medical school. "The university's a financial parasite. It didn't pay attention to our needs for twenty years."

These transfers were not new, preventing the medical center, and particularly the hospital, from building reserves to weather the challenging times that were coming.[34]* A particularly onerous extraction, as the hospital executives saw it, was a $20 million mandated "contribution" from the hospital to general university funds in 1986,[23] "to pay for the deficits in the English department," as one of the medical department administrators described one of the purposes of the transfers.[36] The transactions continued in subsequent years in "the $3.5 to $5 million range," according to O'Brien.[37] This was money that he and his associates wanted to invest in the hospital and its clinical programs.

The university president was heard to say, "I was surprised that I got away with it so easily." One of the veterans on the medical faculty commented that this reflected the "lovely Georgetown spirit," that no one would have challenged the president.[10]

---

*"These types of transfers of funds were taking place in at least several other academic medical centers at that time to my knowledge, not just at Georgetown," explains Stuart Bondurant, executive dean at the Georgetown medical center.[35]

Why the Medical Center Developed Financial Trouble

Despite the administrative changes that his predecessors had instituted, Bloem and others found that the medical center suffered from a malfunctioning infrastructure.[22,34,38,39] It lacked local control of most administrative functions, which prevented the hospital from responding quickly and creatively to its problems. Finance (including general ledger, accounts payable, and audit), information technology, engineering, maintenance of buildings, human resources, and labor negotiations, among other tasks, were all controlled at the university level. Both the university and the medical center once had budget committees, but Griffith dissolved the medical center's committee when he became executive dean.

"Accounting was not very good," Bloem said, "worse than at anywhere I'd worked."[22] With all financial reporting from the hospital, medical school, nursing school, full-time practices, and research programs integrated in one office, it was exceedingly difficult to know which entity was losing and which was making money, how much money was involved, and where the money was going.[36]

Hospital income, on which the school depended,[40] began to fall, the faculty did not develop the grants as quickly as planned,[40] philanthropy to support research did not materialize,[40] and the pharmaceutical company that would use half of Griffith's new research building went bankrupt.[8] Most of the money for the new laboratory building had been borrowed and the medical center, assigned the costs of the interest and amortization, was then left with the expense of retrofitting the space that the defunct company would have occupied.

Then there was the costly closing of the dental school during the last half of the 1980s,[1] widely acknowledged to be the right thing to do, but for which Griffith "took a lot of heat."[12,28] The school had been losing money for years, it had no practice plan to collect money for clinical services, and its faculty had few grants. Consequently, the university had to charge a high tuition, which, along with decreasing interest in dentistry as a career, reduced the number and quality of the students. With the school going through the process of shutting down and the alumni complaining that their alma mater was being closed, "its problems were distracting us from other issues," remembers Griffith.[1]

As the dental school was phased out, the amount of tuition decreased and then stopped, but the medical center still had to maintain the build-ings and pay the faculty until they left or retired.[22] This could be expensive since Georgetown's salary commitments at the time were quite generous, and the salaries of investigators and clinicians were never lowered if they lost grants or their practices decreased.[22] On retirement, tenured faculty throughout the university, including the medical school, were annually paid the highest salary they had ever earned. When they died, their sur-vivors received one payment of a year's salary.

Griffith and his staff tried unsuccessfully to decrease the tenure ex-pense.[22,28] He formed a committee on medical school tenure and compen-sation that concluded that salaries, particularly in the basic sciences, should be reduced to a "base" when grants went away. This would decrease the amount paid when faculty members retired. Despite the school's having de-veloped an incentive-driven compensation scheme for the clinicians, when highly paid specialists retired, the school had to pay them the maximum yearly salary they had ever earned, which could be as much as $500,000 per year.

An attempt to define the financial obligations of tenure at the Medical Center greatly angered the medical school faculty as well as other faculty members, who feared that the university might apply a similar model in their schools.[41] A group of faculty filed a class-action suit that the university lawyers thought Georgetown could win. However, rather than face the publicity and internal divisiveness that a prolonged action might create, the university rescinded the policy. The expensive tenure plan continued, leading one member of the senior faculty to say, "Financially, it didn't make sense."[17]

The continuing financial problems had frozen Griffith's plans to im-prove Georgetown medicine's academic power and were challenging his ability to successfully administer the medical center. "This was not the time," one of the basic scientists said, "to have an amateur running the place." The majority of those in the medical school polled by the faculty council in 1996 rebuked Griffith's leadership, a marked change from the enthusiasm that greeted what he was accomplishing during the first half of his tenure.[41]

"I felt burned out," Griffith explains. "I wanted uniqueness and quality, but the university wasn't set on where it wanted to go."[1] He left in Au-gust.[41] Milton Corn, Griffith's predecessor as dean, said, "John's goals were very high. He wanted to model the school on Duke, but this was inappropriate for Georgetown. Duke had much better research, supported by the strong influence it had in North Carolina, much greater than we had in the district."[10]

Soon after Griffith left, Nelson Ford, the medical center's chief operating and financial officer, resigned, thereby depriving the medical center of another of its senior executives. In the absence of adequate financial or organizational systems,[34] Ford "carried it all around in his head," which would predictably cause trouble for his successor. Furthermore, research dean Alan Faden said, "financial projections presented to the university were at times unrealistically optimistic, thereby diminishing confidence in the medical center when targets were not met."[7] "With Griffith's downfall," a former chairman said, "all the dollar problems were attributed to him."[18]*

New Leadership

The next executive vice president of health sciences and executive dean of the school of medicine was Dr. Sam Wiesel, a spine surgeon, chairman of the department of orthopedic surgery, and chairman of the faculty's prac-

---

*The medical center's financial woes would spread into other parts of the university. At the highly respected Georgetown Law School, the dean Judith Areen, reputed to be a dissident voice in the cabinet of Father Leo O'Donovan, who had succeeded Timothy Healy as Georgetown president in 1989, had been objecting to the university's taxing other schools to support the losses in medicine, according to *The Washington Post* and several members of the medical faculty and administration.[22,42-44]

On April 9, 1998, the *Post* reported that the university would not renew Areen's contract when her current term as dean ended a year later.[44] This action brought strong protests from students and faculty in the law school.[45] Alumni donors withdrew nearly $4 million in pledges,[46] and some members of the law school's board of visitors resigned.[46] Ten days after the university had announced that it would not renew Areen's contract, president O'Donovan agreed to reappoint her for another term.[47]

Caught up in this conflict was Michael Kelly, the university's senior vice president and chief operating officer. "My job," Kelly explains, "was to be vice president for the whole university."[15] The executive vice presidents for medicine and law and the provost, who has authority for the other academic departments on the main campus,[48] report directly to the president.[49] Each guards this prerogative zealously and helps to explain why Georgetown's senior administration remains decentralized.[50]

According to the *Post*, Kelly was "behind the effort to oust Areen because she had resisted his efforts to gain more control over law school funds to help close a huge deficit at Georgetown Medical Center."[51] Kelly resigned on April 30, thereby removing his strong advocacy for the medical school at the university level.[51] "Michael took the fall for O'Donovan's decision about Judy," one of the medical professors said.[6]

Kelly's successor was John DeGioia, who upon O'Donovan's retirement in June 2001, would become the university president.[52]

tice plan. One of the chairmen called him "a physician's physician."[6] As Wiesel puts it, "they replaced the cognitive Griffith with the non-cognitive me."[17] The turmoil at the time had prevented Georgetown from conducting the usual national search for someone to fill this senior position.[7]

When Wiesel became the executive vice president, the medical center's CEO was Kenneth Bloem, previously CEO of the Stanford University Hospital. Georgetown University president Leo O'Donovan had invited Bloem onto the university board in the spring of 1996 "to provide oversight in view of my experience."[22] Bloem is, in the words of a former senior university official, "the charismatic son of a preacher. A very impressive man."[15]

Bloem and Wiesel split the leadership.[38] Functionally, Wiesel became the chief academic officer and Bloem the chief business officer of the medical center.[8,41] Wiesel led the medical school and the clinicians, while Bloem ran the hospital and liaised with the board of directors. "We worked in one office and shared one staff," Bloem said. "We were, in effect, co-CEOs and looked on both jobs as short-term rescue efforts."[24]

When they started, "Sam and Ken didn't know how bad the trouble was," remembers Dr. Richard Goldberg, the chairman of psychiatry and successor to Wiesel as president of the medical school's faculty practice plan.[9] Since finances were still centralized in the university, understanding where the losses were coming from was very difficult. "Georgetown was in a financial management mess," said Michael O'Boyle, the chief financial officer at MedStar Health, which would buy the Georgetown University Hospital in 2000. "The systems were so convoluted that it was impossible to follow the flow of funds."[53]*

Despite the advice from consultants[36,54] and Bloem's and Wiesel's best efforts, the losses, though somewhat reduced, continued, and Georgetown's board of directors finally ordered that the hospital be sold and the practice plan separated.[2] Many members of the faculty heard that the directors even considered closing the whole medical enterprise, including the medical school, if a solution could not be found.[19,27,31,32,36,55-57] Some university officials and members of the board considered the medical center "a terrible burden"[27] and "wanted it to go away."[36] As for the hospital, one of its executives said, "Though we had a few good quarters, we could never get ahead of the curve."[34]

---

*O'Boyle is now chief operating officer of the Cleveland Clinic Foundation.

Bloem had had less than two years to try to reverse the losses* when the university reassigned him from operational control of the hospital to developing the means of selling the hospital and practice plan. Dr. Paul Katz, chairman of the department of medicine, then became chief operating officer of the medical center with particular responsibility for the faculty. Working with a consultant, Katz, whose position of chief operating officer was a new creation, described his charge as "developing a turnaround plan to prepare the hospital for acquisition, not for a merger."[6] Katz reported to Bloem and Wiesel, who concentrated on strategic planning, particularly the sale of the hospital.[18]

Finding a Buyer

Kenneth Bloem now met with President O'Donovan, John ("Jack") DeGioia, then the university's senior vice president, and the directors to decide once and for all what to do with Georgetown's financially ailing hospital.[22] "Panic was setting in," remembered one of the medical center administrators. "The university had been oblivious to our problems, and when they learned about them, they became punitive," by taking funds from reserves that the departments had accumulated for development.[32,36]†

The directors by this time were increasingly worried that the medical center losses would deplete Georgetown's endowment of $703.6 million[58] when selling the hospital was being considered in fiscal 1999.[59]‡ The losses were also beginning to affect the ability of the university to borrow money at a favorable rate.[61]

Not wanting to lose any more money through the hospital or practice plan, Georgetown's leadership chose to rid itself of both of its clinical en-

---

*The new owners of the hospital would take five years to produce a surplus.

† "Reserves were not 'taken'—they were used to cover medical center losses," one of the medical center officials wrote me upon reviewing the manuscript. "The university worked very hard to turn around the enterprise fiscally before concluding that it was better to find a clinical partner. Logic and experience, not panic, led to the decision that selling the clinical enterprise would be Georgetown's best course. Reasonable people can debate whether that was a correct conclusion, but the deliberation that led to it is pretty clear."[58]

‡ By 2005, Georgetown University's endowment was $741 million, which ranked it seventy-eighth among the nation's colleges and universities.[60] The medical school's portion of this was about $90 million, which generates annually about $5 million of unrestricted income.[17] Despite its founding almost two centuries previously, the university had not started raising money seriously until the 1980s.[38]

tities.[9,12] To avoid paying further for future medical center losses, faculty members in other schools within the university also favored this approach. As one observer of the process commented, "The culture just didn't have the appetite to risk capital or further indebtedness, nor did the directors have the resolve to do otherwise."

Borrowing to support the medical center was not a possibility. The university's debt/endowment ratio was a precarious 1:1.[38]* The university would merge the hospital and the practice group with, or sell them to, one of the major medical centers. The question was no longer whether to sell but to whom to sell.[31] Some considered that even a for-profit company might be acceptable, as it had been at George Washington three years earlier.[24]

This was not the first time that the university had contemplated selling the hospital.[23,28,29] In the mid-1980s, when the hospital was making money,[28] the university leaders thought they could increase the endowment by selling it for $250 to $300 million.[23] The hospital executives also proposed a modified leveraged buyout in which the hospital would be reconstituted as a separate not-for-profit corporation and would pay the university annually an amount equal to the interest that the proceeds of a private sale would generate. Neither proposal was adopted. John Griffith opposed each partially because, it was said, the executive vice president could no longer coordinate all the parts of the Georgetown medical center.[23]

Bloem thought that "the ideal solution [in the late 1990s] was for Johns Hopkins to take us over."[22] As Bloem saw it, Georgetown offered to the Hopkins clinical enterprise the opportunity to directly enter the Washington market. Georgetown could provide respected programs in health policy, law, biomedical ethics, and cancer and assist Hopkins in establishing itself in the nation's capital. The National Institutes of Health (NIH), from which Hopkins medical science receives much support, was not far away in Bethesda.

In 1997, Bloem and Wiesel jointly approached Dr. Edward Miller, the dean of the Hopkins school of medicine and CEO of Johns Hopkins Medicine.[17] The Georgetown team suggested that Hopkins take over the hospital and medical school and create, in effect, "Johns Hopkins Medicine at Georgetown."[17]

Miller remembers the discussions:[63]

* As it also was at George Washington University.[62]

Georgetown approached us for a relationship with Johns Hopkins Medicine. We had several meetings in quiet places that were far enough apart but relatively close. We wanted an international presence in DC. There were possible cancer links with their Lombardi Cancer Center and some potential connections in basic science. We knew about their clinical problems, particularly in cardiology and cardiac surgery, and suspected that they may have seen us as a lifeline.

The discussions went quite a long way, but we couldn't understand where their basic sciences were, couldn't figure out where they were financially, and were concerned about the Jesuit restrictions. Would both faculties favor or not favor this, and what about the faculty appointments? Eventually we decided that we didn't want to take on the liabilities and that it just didn't make sense for us.

Particularly troubling to the Hopkins leadership was the perception that Georgetown University was sending a message to the medical faculty that clinical practice and research were less significant missions than teaching the students.[39] "At the end of the day," Bloem said, "Hopkins concluded it was too much of a risk."[24]

When the Hopkins merger failed, Georgetown considered some of the national Catholic hospital-owning systems. Bloem also had preliminary talks with Knox Singleton, the CEO of Inova, the not-for-profit company based in Northern Virginia that owned the successful Fairfax Hospital where Georgetown students and residents trained. "Inova appeared financially stronger than any hospital or hospital group in the area other than Hopkins," Bloem concluded. "It was making real profits, had strong managed care contracts, owned real estate in a rapidly growing, wealthy region, and wanted stronger teaching programs."[24] The negotiations with Inova, however, progressed slowly and inconclusively. Eventually, the Georgetown directors rejected Inova's proposal,[17] which was seen as a "low-ball offer"[15] and "a draconian solution."[9] Discussions with for-profit hospital-owning corporations were stymied, in part, over issues related to Catholic policies.[9] As a former Georgetown dean noted, "the Jesuit mission wouldn't allow it to be sold to a for-profit."[19]

With none of these overtures going very far, it was beginning to look as if "no one wanted to buy it," remembers Dr. Stuart Bondurant,* then a consultant to DeGioia, the senior vice president of the university.[2]

*Bondurant would later twice serve as interim executive vice president and executive dean of the medical center from December 2002 to July 2003 and from the summer of 2004 until April 2007. Counting Bondurant twice, Georgetown would have five permanent or interim executive vice presidents from 2000 to 2007.

The one institution that showed more than passing interest in acquiring the Georgetown University Hospital was MedStar Health, a not-for-profit hospital-owning corporation whose flagship is the Washington Hospital Center, the largest hospital in the city. MedStar also owned four community hospitals in Baltimore and the National Rehabilitation Hospital in Washington.

Just when Georgetown thought it would have "to pay someone to take over the hospital,"[9] MedStar made a generous offer to pay the university $80 million at once plus an additional $15 million for the rights to certain other clinical facilities. Although faculty hoped that this money would be directed toward research and education,[57] the funds "were entirely consumed by existing and future medical center debt and transaction costs," according to Laura Cavender, Georgetown's executive director of communications for the medical center.[3]*

Because MedStar was obtaining a hospital that had lost $61.9 million in fiscal year 1999,[3]† Georgetown observers wondered why the purchaser was so generous. "MedStar, in retrospect, likely overbid," believes Richard Goldberg, "because they were so eager to have an academic hospital in their system."[9]‡ Many at Georgetown felt that of all the potential buyers, MedStar was the most likely to support the academic mission.[31]§

Under the terms of the "clinical partnership," MedStar Health would acquire and operate the Georgetown clinical enterprise, consisting of the university hospital, the Faculty Practice Group, two outpatient satellites, and a network of community physician practices.[66] The university leased to MedStar at $1 per year for ninety-nine years, plus a renewal option of fifty-one years, the land under the hospital, the Pasquerilla Healthcare Center, where the doctors see their outpatients, the Lombardi clinical building for cancer patients, and two parking garages. The two parties developed three

*The university incurred significant expenses just to complete the deal. These included retiring $89 million of debt on clinical facilities, providing one-time payments to tenured clinical faculty, continuing to offer tuition benefits to employees transferring to MedStar, purchasing outside professional services needed to complete the partnership, supplying transitional services during the first year of the partnership, and reducing the size and scope of medical center administration during and after the transition.[3]

†In the same year, the medical school lost $22.2 million.[9] Georgetown prefers to assign this to the "medical center's research and educational activities."[64]

‡See chapter 9 for MedStar's reasons for buying Georgetown.

§"The Washington Hospital Center at least claims to be an academic institution," said a former member of the Georgetown faculty. "Inova does not."[65]

agreements that established their new relationship: the long-term lease, the asset purchase, and the academic affiliation.[67]

Bloem Leaves

As soon as the letter of intent between the university and MedStar was signed, Kenneth Bloem left Georgetown. With MedStar and its own executives about to take charge, "there was no place for me," he was heard to say.

Kenneth Bloem's efforts to institute fundamental changes at Georgetown had been unavailing. "I was led to believe that I would take over the administrative and financial functions as they related to the hospital," Bloem said, "but I never could."[22] O'Donovan had told Bloem that he would change the structure. "Didn't happen. The place had structural shackles."[22] Others confirm that O'Donovan, though saying all the right things about advancing medicine at Georgetown, did not always follow through effectively on what his faculty and medical administration advised.[7] Bloem's experience had confirmed his belief that "academic hospitals must control the administrative levers."[24] The board refused an external review that Bloem recommended. "They didn't want me meddling."[22]

With Georgetown and MedStar having completed the "dating process" and preparing a preliminary letter of intent, Bloem and O'Donovan decided that Bloem could move on since he had accomplished most of his charge. Others could complete the due diligence process and write the final agreements leading to the marriage of MedStar and the Georgetown University Hospital. MedStar's ownership of the hospital meant that its management would now be in the hands of an experienced organization, better able to deal with its challenges than had been the university's administration.[24]

The Georgetown engagement had been frustrating for Ken Bloem. "I found myself in the middle of a vortex and became," he believes, "the sacrificial lamb."[24] So Bloem left Georgetown three years after he had arrived.

MedStar Takes Over

MedStar installed Dr. Joy Drass as the hospital president. Drass, a critical care internist, is a graduate of Georgetown's medical school and the Wharton School at the University of Pennsylvania (M.B.A.). Before taking her current job, she was a senior administrator at MedStar's Washington Hospital Center, where she began working as an intern in 1973. Drass's participation in the due diligence phase of the merger made her "a strong and unique individual," believed Kenneth Samet, MedStar's president and COO, capable of rescuing the hospital from its financial morass.[68]

Initially, with its annual loss then $38 million, MedStar hoped that the Georgetown University Hospital under Drass's administration would break even, before interest payments, by the end of the third year.[68,69] This occurred, but it took five years before the hospital made a profit (including interest.)[68] By then the hospital would grow to accommodate as many as 400 patients, about 200 more than before MedStar took over. The average daily census is now about 350 patients, not counting those remaining in the hospital for less than 24 hours.[67]

How did Drass and MedStar do it? "We stabilized operations and improved services, improved revenue cycles, and managed care contracts," she explains. "We maintained a consistent message and stayed focused on our priorities. Strategy informed all our decisions. We used capital dollars and space as metrics."[67] The takeover forced Drass and her associates "to understand funds flows that weren't understood before because of all the deals," she said. "No one could remember them all. The commingling of funds was a mess."[67]

The clinical programs in each department are expected to break even.[70] The absence of a tax helps them do so. Departments may retain surpluses, but the money must be spent for clinical projects, not for research, and be approved by the hospital's administration.[70] "Our agreement with the university," Drass explains, "specified that the university would fund research and MedStar would fund clinical activities."[71] The agreement also provided that when a surplus generated by MedStar at the hospital and practice plan exceeds a certain value, the university will receive some of it for academic purposes. As of the fall of 2006, Drass would say, "the 'gain sharing provision' hasn't been tripped yet."[71] The hospital, however, has assigned two floors in one of its buildings on the Georgetown campus to the medical school to accommodate clinical research programs.[71]

Why couldn't Georgetown have done it? "They didn't have MedStar's clinical operations experience and expertise," said Drass.[67] Billing and collection were primitive,[65,72] dismal in the hospital* though somewhat better in the practice plan. Reimbursement from managed care contracts, which

---

*The average number of days in accounts receivable was about 130 at its worst.[6]

had been consistently accepted at uneconomically low levels under university management,[18,24,28,72-75] could now be negotiated for all the MedStar hospitals and doctors than just for Georgetown alone.[17] The hospital's finances were also helped by MedStar's not having to support the central university or the medical school—MedStar no longer paid the dean a portion of the doctors' practice.[17,57] Of course, these changes made balancing the school's budget more difficult.

"In today's difficult health care environment, hospitals must demonstrate adaptability in order to remain viable in a fiercely competitive market," Drass added. "The ability to respond to changes in the market is essential to growth and success in a very turbulent health care marketplace. Change naturally requires institutions to be flexible and nimble if they want to succeed. Making decisions takes a long time, which is appropriate in a university atmosphere where the mission is to foster and embrace knowledge and consensus, but it is not effective in the health care environment, which is in chaos every day. You need to move very fast."[76]

The differences between MedStar's and the university's style of management evoked several comments:[8,70,77-80]

- "The university couldn't make the tough decisions the medical center needed. The academic mindset interfered. Decision making by committee doesn't work, especially when the ship is sinking."
- University decision making is "very process oriented" and involves "lots of collegiality with lots of people involved in making decisions," whereas MedStar is "a very business and operationally oriented place, focused on outcomes, performance measures, and the bottom line, like a for-profit."
- "MedStar governs with corporate, top-down, centralized decision making, not diffusely as universities do."
- "We didn't have enough experienced people in finance. In the critical period from 1992 to 1996, we just weren't minding the store."
- "It was the intertwining of inadequately developed financial data between the hospital, practice plan, and university."
- "Georgetown at the time had two fatal flaws, ignorance with arrogance."

Until the end of the 1980s, voluntary faculty admitted most of the patients to the Georgetown University Hospital.[23] John Griffith changed this by actively recruiting full-time clinicians so that by 1995, they admitted 85 percent of the patients.[17] At the same time, he discouraged members of the voluntary faculty, on whom the hospital had long depended to fill the beds,[10,17] from admitting patients.[10,23,26,81]

By the time of the sale, the leaders of the clinical departments were having increasing difficulty convincing physicians and surgeons to practice at Georgetown.[56] Not many voluntary physicians now considered Georgetown their home, and few could be persuaded to admit their patients there.[39] With MedStar resources, the physician shortage was relieved in several departments, but one effect of this effort had been to produce a clinical faculty that emphasizes practice over research.[56]

Most of the medical staff are particularly pleased that Drass and her team have markedly improved the aging physical plant the company had inherited.[53,78] In addition to buying expensive equipment,[72] the hospital made several low-profile investments, such as replacing all the Gurney stretchers and infusion pumps, to the approval of the medical staff.[55] MedStar improved the quality and morale of the nonprofessional workforce, seen previously as "difficult."[54]

Six years out, many,[2,7,32,55,56,70,74,78,82,83] though not all,[29,84] of those now or formerly in the academic clinical departments believe that selling the hospital to MedStar was wise and that the hospital is better managed under MedStar than when the university owned it.* "It brought calmness, a different way of thinking," said Michael Pentecost, the chairman of radiology from 1996 to 2005.[55] As Joseph Verbalis, the interim chair of medicine, says, "We're better off than if we were owned by a for-profit. But if the five-year plan hadn't worked, we might all have had to leave Georgetown and move to other academic medical centers."[56]

Although many praise Joy Drass and her team for improving the hospital and reversing its losses and find her "easy to deal with,"[56] some find her administration less than ideal for a university hospital. Alan Faden, the veteran Georgetown neuroscientist, believes, "The leadership of MedStar has not sufficiently supported the academic clinical enterprise."[7]† Kimford

---

*Including John McDaniel, MedStar's CEO. "I am very proud of the tremendous turnaround at Georgetown in all respects. It may well be one of the greatest ever for an academic medical center, which I attribute (modestly speaking) to their being a part of our integrated health care delivery system."[85]

†"This is not true. MedStar has consistently supported the academic clinical enterprise by hiring new physician recruits and enhancing programs through the purchase of new medical technologies," a MedStar executive replies.[68]

Meador, the former neurology chairman and, admittedly, not a Drass supporter, says "she is inappropriate to lead an academic center because she has no vision about academic goals. The medical school has little leverage against her and has lost control of its clinical faculty because it has no money, and Joy primarily cares about money." As for her management style, Meador says, "Joy makes decisions on what is fed to her and never changes her mind because that might be seen as a sign of weakness. It's a very insular and hierarchical management style that does not translate well to an academic institution."[86]

Robert Martuza, chairman of neurosurgery at Georgetown from 1991 to 2000 and now chairman of the department at the Massachusetts General Hospital, says, "As for Georgetown's having no choice, people always have choices. Georgetown could have been the major hospital in the nation's capital. It takes decades to build an academic medical center, but it can go downhill in just two years. It's a sad story."[84]

In Alan Faden's opinion, "MedStar's taken Georgetown and transitioned it to an efficient, largely non-academic, hospital,"[7] and in the view of one of the former chairmen, "It's now a good community hospital without full services."[12] "Not true," replies MedStar. "In many instances the technologies, services, and procedures offered at Georgetown cannot be found anywhere in the area. Peripheral nerve surgery, small bowel transplant, CyberKnife were first offered at Georgetown on the East Coast."[68]

Georgetown Cardiology and Cardiac Surgery

There was a time, several decades ago, when Georgetown was a major force in the diagnosis and treatment of heart disease and the training of practicing and academic cardiologists. In the 1960s and 1970s, Georgetown had "prestige, location, and Harvey and Hufnagel," as Dr. Stuart Seides, a cardiologist and veteran of the local wars, remembers.[43]* Harvey was Dr. W. Proctor Harvey, the chief of cardiology, who had developed a world-renowned training program based, to a great extent, on his skill in teaching physical diagnosis, an important diagnostic method particularly in the specialty's earlier days before more advanced techniques had been

---

*Seides, who has been a member of both the GW and Georgetown medical faculties, trained in cardiology at Georgetown, where he had also been chief medical resident.

developed. His surgical colleague was Dr. Charles Hufnagel, who invented the first satisfactory way of treating leaking aortic valves.*

Then, according to Seides and others, Georgetown made "one mistake after another."[16,23,28,43,65,81,88-91]

- *Restricted use of catheterization laboratory.* Georgetown continued to limit use of the catheterization laboratory to cardiologists who were salaried members of the full-time staff, just as GW and many other university hospitals did, thereby driving the increasingly busy voluntary cardiologists to do their work at other hospitals.
- *Features of Harvey's leadership.* Harvey's dominance in physical diagnosis, which was largely confined to auscultation, limited the development of the newer techniques in cardiology such as echocardiography, nuclear cardiology, and electrophysiology.
- *Referral practices.* During and after Harvey's directorship, the clinical leadership continued to follow a faulty philosophy, common in academic medical centers, that patients would come to the university hospital because "we're here; send us your patients" and eschewed more specific efforts to develop the clinical practice.
- *Slow acceptance of new surgical techniques.* When the coronary artery bypass graft operation (CABG) was developed, Hufnagel—he was not alone in this—did not embrace the new technique. By the time the CABG had been widely accepted, Hufnagel was close to retirement. His successors did not acquire the reputation in the community that he had had. Competition had stiffened as surgeons trained in coronary surgery, like Dr. Jorge Garcia at the Washington Hospital Center, became increasingly well known for their skills and availability. Hufnagel also resisted installing valve prostheses other than his own.

In the early 1980s Georgetown tried to recapture some of its luster in heart disease. The dean at the time appointed specialists in this field as

---

*Called aortic insufficiency or aortic regurgitation in medspeak. In 1952, Hufnagel inserted a prosthesis that successfully reduced the amount of blood leaking back into the left ventricle because of a faulty native valve.[87] He placed his device in the descending aorta without opening the heart. With the development of the heart-lung machine, which allowed surgeons to work directly on the heart, Hufnagel's procedure was superseded by direct repair or replacement of the valve. Working continuously at Georgetown, Hufnagel continued to make important contributions to cardiac surgery for many years.

chairmen of medicine, surgery, and radiology.[10] By now, however, cardiology clinical services were "so far behind"[10] that by the time Dr. Bernard Gersh arrived from the Mayo Clinic as cardiology division chief (1993–98), admissions to the hospital and outpatient visits to the full-time cardiologists were, according to Gersh, "incredibly low. Many full-time and private practice physicians had left Georgetown and were working quite happily at the Washington Hospital Center, Fairfax, and other regional centers, including Suburban and the Washington Adventist hospitals."[92] Gersh thought the medical center "schizophrenic" about how to deal with the voluntary faculty. "We wouldn't give them offices, and they had to pay too much for parking. You can't make them leave and then expect them to come back, even as volunteers."[92]*

"It had become very hard to practice cardiology at Georgetown and advise patients to go there," said former Georgetown cardiologist Manuel Cerqueira. Wanting to stay in Washington if possible, he spoke with the chairman of medicine and chief of cardiology at George Washington. "That didn't seem like a stable situation either," so he responded to an offer from the Cleveland Clinic, where he is now chairman of molecular and functional imaging in the renowned heart center there.[42,93]

James Cox was the chief of cardiac surgery whom Georgetown hired in 1997. Described by colleagues as "an inspired leader," "a true academic,[81] and "a creative clinical scientist," Cox had developed the "MAZE" operation to treat cardiac arrhythmias while a faculty member at Washington University in St. Louis. Although arrhythmia surgery was a small-volume practice, Cox expanded the Georgetown service in coronary and valve surgery so that the number of procedures using cardiopulmonary bypass increased from about two hundred to six hundred cases per year.[65]

But Cox encountered several serious problems while trying to build a successful program at Georgetown. Although he had been told that the hospital was losing about $15 million per year when he was recruited, analysis soon revealed that the correct figure was $85 million per year. "We didn't know this when we hired you," Sam Wiesel explained, "so we can't hire all the people you need."[65] Consequently, the $6 million he had been promised to build the program never materialized although Wiesel insisted

---

*Gersh is now professor of medicine and associate chair for academic affairs and faculty development in the division of cardiovascular diseases in the Mayo College of Medicine.

that Cox receive the salary that he had been promised when he was hired.[65] Cox's clinical work was hampered by having to rely on less well-trained general surgical residents. Georgetown then had none of the more experienced cardiac surgical fellows.[91]

When Cox returned to the operating room three months after having both of his knees replaced, many members of his nursing and other supporting staff members had left or been laid off as the hospital tried to reduce its costs. Unable to stand on his feet continuously for the time needed for the operations and frustrated by Georgetown's inability to provide what he thought was needed "to assure that the surgery we perform is safe," Cox resigned from the university in 2000—after his tenure was bought out—and retired from practicing surgery.[65]

One of the bulwarks in the department of medicine who left was Kenneth ("Kenny") Kent, M.D., Ph.D., a nationally known academic cardiologist who arrived at Georgetown in 1981 after spending much of his early career at the NIH. While he directed the catheterization laboratories at Georgetown from 1983 to 1990,[94] the medical services that he and his colleagues provided their patients accounted for as much as $20 million per year. Kent also supported the salaries of trainees and other associates from his clinical income.[23] The hospital accommodated his needs by buying most of the equipment Kent requested. He left in 1990, however, when Griffith began rejecting his requests and actively discouraging physicians in private practice like him to remain unless they converted to full-time status, which he refused to do. Kent and his colleagues left Georgetown and formed a private professional corporation that became very large and successful. Based at the Washington Hospital Center, their clinical practices added to the already flourishing cardiac program there.[88]* "After that," says hospital CEO Chuck O'Brien, "we couldn't compete in cardiology."[23]

When MedStar took over in 2000, "adult cardiac surgery at Georgetown was functionally closed because of physician and staff losses," Joy Drass said. "We tried to build a program with surgeons from the Washington Hospital Center, but there was too much competition in the area."[76]

---

*Ironically, it was Kent whom MedStar dispatched back to Georgetown as director of cardiology from 2000 to 2003. When Georgetown's cardiac surgery program closed, Kent left Georgetown for the second time to become chief of cardiology at Suburban Hospital in Bethesda, Maryland, where the National Heart, Lung, and Blood Institute is developing a comprehensive clinical and research program in cardiology and cardiac surgery.[88]

These disheartening efforts to build strong medical and surgical cardiac programs at Georgetown led the physiologist Martin Morad to advise that Georgetown emphasize basic research in the field rather than directly competing with the Hospital Center.[89]

"I was asked to set up a cardiac surgical satellite at Georgetown," said Dr. Paul Corso, the senior surgeon of the largest cardiac surgical practice in Washington. He and his colleagues, who are based at the Hospital Center, operate on about 2,300 patients annually. "I had to convince the doctors who used to refer to Georgetown to send their patients there again. Couldn't do it. They weren't willing to come back no matter what we did. The university had so irritated them in the past. It would obviously make no economic sense for MedStar to send patients from the Hospital Center there."[81]*

The Georgetown hospital estimated that it could only operate a profitable medical and surgical cardiac program if the number of surgical cases exceeded four hundred per year.[88] When the volume failed to reach three hundred per year by 2003, MedStar closed the program.[67,73,81,88,95]† "We couldn't move business from Northern Virginia, and 9/11 had a negative impact on the international business," said Kenneth Samet, MedStar's president.[96] Without the assurance that cardiac services could grow enough to succeed, MedStar was unwilling to invest the capital needed for a fully contemporary cardiology program. The hospital decided to concentrate its limited resources on those programs with a record of success at Georgetown, such as transplantation of liver and other gastrointestinal organs, complex interventional GI services, oncology, neurosurgery, and vascular surgery.[67,88]‡ The pediatric cardiac surgeons had left in 2000.[73]§

*Corso understands this from his position as a member of the board of directors of MedStar.

†Transferring most of Georgetown's cardiac programs to the Washington Hospital Center has been one of the few decisions directly affecting professional services at Georgetown that was made at the MedStar corporate level by John McDaniel, the chief executive officer, and Kenneth Samet, the president and chief operating officer.[81] "Joy had to accept this," said one of the chairmen.[95]

‡Dean of medical education Ray Mitchell says that the Georgetown hospital is looking more and more like a specialty hospital "like the Hospital for Special Surgery in New York City," which specializes in the treatment of patients with orthopedic and rheumatic diseases.[72]

§Consequently, the pediatric cardiologist at Georgetown had to send his patients needing operations elsewhere. He favored children's hospitals in other cities over the Children's National Medical Center in Washington despite an agreement that required that DC Children's would be the "provider of choice" for Georgetown pediatric cardiac surgery.[97] This presented Joy Drass with a problem since Washington Children's implied that it would remove one of its surgeons from Georgetown, which depended on him for general pediatric surgery, unless the cardiologist referred his patients to DC

While some thought that closing cardiology was "the right business decision,"[72] others disputed the wisdom of doing so,[7,29,55,70] Michael Pentecost,
the former chairman of radiology, called it "very distressing, a decision of
pivotal importance," and wonders whether the action may, in the future,
prove to be unwise.[55] Another chairman commented, "MedStar didn't bring
most of us into the decision to close cardiac surgery. But that's MedStar's
way. When they see something's not working, they do something about it
and quickly."[70]

Reducing the role of cardiology at Georgetown angered those with strong
attachments to the specialty there. "The decision created quite a furor,"
Paul Corso remembers.[81] The cardiac surgery experience has convinced one
member of the senior faculty that "MedStar wants the Washington Hospital
Center to become the center of its academics. But this won't happen because
the private practitioners are so strong there. They don't have the academic
point of view."*

In medical cardiology, Bernard Gersh went back to the Mayo Clinic in
1998. "I wanted to return to an academic life, and by then I'd gotten the
chief business out of my system. I certainly enjoyed much of my time at
Georgetown but was not optimistic that the fundamental financial problems affecting the institution could be corrected."[92] After Gersh left, cardiology would be directed by a series of chiefs, none of whom remained in
the position for long.

"Morale was dropping, everybody was leaving so there was no one to
talk to. It wasn't fun anymore," Dr. Allen Solomon in the electrophysiology
(EP) laboratory remembers. "They wanted us to move EP to the Washington Hospital Center. We'd always competed with the group there; they
wouldn't speak to us. Didn't look good."[98] So Solomon and his colleague
Dr. Cynthia Tracy moved to George Washington. Georgetown failed to
maintain an active EP service after their departure.[99] By the summer of
2006, only five cardiologists were based at Georgetown University Hospital,
"a shell of a division," Solomon called it.[98]

Children's. When the cardiologist continued to refer outside Washington, Drass dismissed him and
replaced him with cardiologists from Children's.[97] The "invasion" from DC Children's caused "much
ill feeling" in the Georgetown pediatrics department.[73]

*Though some did earlier in their careers. "Quite a few of the doctors there were faculty, at
Georgetown, George Washington, and elsewhere who decided that private practice was what they
wanted to do. They're not interested in having the Hospital Center converted into the kind of places
they left," said a former chairman.

Georgetown cardiologists who perform cardiac catheterizations do the procedures at the Washington Hospital Center. With the reduction in cardiac services at Georgetown, patients who come to the hospital with serious heart problems or develop them while in the hospital are transferred by helicopter to the Washington Hospital Center.[88]

In the summer of 2006, MedStar and Georgetown, which made a significant financial commitment,[38] recruited Dr. Leslie Miller to direct a unique combined medical cardiology program at the Washington Hospital Center and Georgetown University Hospital. Miller came from the University of Minnesota, where he held the analogous position of chief of cardiology. Heart failure is his particular clinical and research interest. "I am enthused about this being a model of the future for an academic program truly partnering with large private hospitals for not only shared clinical programs, but education and research," writes Miller. "I came to try to forge that integration and seek and use the best of both programs to create a dominant cardiovascular program."[100]

Surgery

Significant town-gown issues greeted Dr. Robert Wallace when he joined Georgetown as chairman of surgery and chief of cardiothoracic surgery in 1980. Wallace planned to develop in Washington, where he had grown up,[16] the type of referral practice he knew from working for much of his career at the Mayo Clinic, where he had become chairman of the department of surgery at the age of thirty-seven. He believed that the hospital could prosper with full-time doctors.[10] At Mayo, which is located in rural Minnesota, most of the patients are referred from other places, some quite distant. Washington medicine did not operate that way. "Practice in Washington is very parochial," he learned. "Integrated group practices as I had known at Mayo were almost nonexistent."[91]

Wallace was not one of John Griffith's favorite faculty members. "Bob spoke for thirty or so surgeons who were the economic engine of the hospital," wrote Dr. Russell Nauta, a trauma surgeon at Georgetown, now at Mt. Auburn Hospital, a Harvard affiliate in Cambridge, Massachusetts. "The disagreements came because his vision, pragmatic and well reasoned, was markedly different than John Griffith's—not because of the economic benefit that Wallace's department brought to the hospital." Wallace accepted that within the practice plan "the wealthier divisions in surgery should subsidize the growth of less wealthy divisions if they derived advantage from having those divisions in the medical center."[101]

Though criticized for favoring his subspecialty—Wallace was chief of cardiac surgery as well as chairman of the department of surgery at Georgetown—he was "the most valuable doctor here," according to Dr. David Pearle, one of the veteran cardiologists and at one time acting chief of the division.[16] Wallace left Georgetown in 1996.

In 2002, the university appointed Dr. Stephen Evans, a general surgeon, to be chairman. Evans had trained and been a member of the junior faculty at Georgetown until 1997, when he moved to George Washington. Following a national search, one of the few the university and MedStar conducted at the time, Evans was brought back to Georgetown to lead the department, which at the time, he says, "was in need of an overhaul."[102]

Since surgery is traditionally a hospital's biggest profit center, MedStar agreed to fund what Evans said was needed to build a strong department. As of June 2006, he had recruited twenty-two new faculty members while losing only three. Four hold the Ph.D. degree and are medical investigators; the rest are practicing surgeons. The department has emphasized the divisions of transplantation, vascular, oncology, and thoracic.[102] Since Georgetown Hospital no longer offers cardiac surgery, operations in this specialty are being performed at the Hospital Center, which is also strong in burns and trauma, specialties that Evans does not plan to emphasize at Georgetown.[102]

To counteract the established referral patterns, Evans has recruited surgeons who perform uncommon, complicated operations. Most community surgeons avoid such operations since results may be poor when a surgeon does only a few per year.* The department's practice has developed so that more than 80 percent of the referrals come from doctors not on the Georgetown staff, frequently surgeons who want an experienced expert to perform the operation. "I work with more than thirty GI docs," Evans said.[102]

Evans has also pushed his faculty and himself to report their experience

---

*Georgetown's team is performing between 150 and 200 pancreatic resections per year, operations that are intricate, time-consuming, and dangerous if performed by surgeons whose volume is not great enough. Evans believes that his group may become a serious competitor with Johns Hopkins, which has a national reputation for pancreatic surgery but has recently lost some of its leading surgeons in this field to retirement or recruitment to other medical schools.[102]

in the medical literature and through courses given at Georgetown and in talks to doctors in the community. He also believes that the department must be productive in clinical and basic research.* It is essential, be believes, that the surgeons he recruits into Washington's saturated market be academic. "We have limited academic competition here," Evans says. "The departments at George Washington and at the Washington Hospital Center are more focused in the clinical realm and less in bench and translational research."[102]

Geographical Problems; Primary Care

The Georgetown clinical enterprise suffers from significant geographic problems.[54] Although located in a choice area of the city, it is distant from the Washington subway system.[77] With a station in the middle of its medical campus, George Washington Hospital is easier to reach, has a busier emergency department, and draws patients from an area with a higher population density.[104,105]† Consequently, Georgetown does not receive many patients with trauma or those in the lower-income groups.[108]

Georgetown is landlocked,[54] with patients from Virginia and the southern suburbs not wanting to cross the Potomac River—"the river's a big divide," said one of Washington's busiest cardiologists[43]—or to come downtown from the northern suburbs. Nevertheless, 65 percent of the hospital's business comes from Virginia and Maryland.[68] Since MedStar took over, admissions from Northern Virginia have grown by 25 to 30 percent.[109] The amount of parking space has long been inadequate for patients and staff.[54] After the MedStar purchase, additional parking spaces were allocated by the university to the clinical enterprise.[68]

"Georgetown found itself not very competitive," observed Ken Bloem when he joined the university board. "The Georgetown hospital and faculty practices were among the weakest in the Washington area. Then there

---

*In the summer of 2006, the department of surgery had one grant from the NIH and had six applications in review.[103]

†GW's emergency department receives about 58,000 visits per year, Georgetown 30,000, Washington Hospital Center 78,000.[106]

Believing that, because of its location, the Georgetown hospital, "doesn't make sense," Alan Miller, CEO of Universal Health Services, which built and owns the new hospital at George Washington, once suggested constructing one hospital for both medical schools on the GW site.[107]

Sam Wiesel agrees that combining the hospitals would permit economies of scale, but "would two losers together equal one winner? Besides, neither party would give up its hospital."[17]

was Hopkins, to which many patients, especially in the northern suburbs, looked for advanced care." As for Georgetown and George Washington, "their medical centers were in the lowest quartile," he said.[22]

Georgetown joined the rush toward forming community clinics and acquiring the practices of primary care physicians in the early and mid- 1990s by forming its Community Practice Network.[77,79] One of the clinics was built in Rockville, Montgomery County, Maryland, and the other in Arlington County in Northern Virginia,[8,77,79] "to stop being stuck on Reservoir Road," as one clinician suggested, referring to the address of the hospital.[110] Each was staffed with about ten primary care physicians. The purpose, as at other academic medical centers, was to increase referrals to the hospital and combat the effects of managed care.[111] Also as elsewhere, the units themselves were loss leaders, unprofitable by themselves.[111] The project was an attempt to counter the difficulty of being a "stand-alone hospital" in Washington.[38] Ironically, not having enough money[38] to spend on the advice consultants were giving at the time saved Georgetown from the losses that followed these failed projects at other centers during the 1990s.[111]

Several of the doctors at these clinics were members of the department of family medicine. Though academically based at Georgetown, the department has never had a clinical presence there.[79] The faculty teach medical students at the Georgetown campus, but its doctors practice at other locations, including at Providence Hospital, a Catholic institution run by the Daughters of Charity and located near Catholic University in Northeast Washington.* The faculty in the department, according to Dr. Jay Siwek, the chairman, "teach in each of the four years. Among our courses are Introduction to Health Care, Ambulatory Care, Evidence Based Medicine, and the family medicine clerkship. We teach in more courses than does any other department."[79]

The creation of these clinics and the hiring of more primary care physicians was part of John Griffith's plan to reorient Georgetown medicine more toward the delivery of primary care and less toward specialty care, the traditional strength of academic medical centers.[11] His enthusiasm for primary care represented a change in emphasis for Griffith. In 1989, according

---

*From the Providence Hospital Web site: "Chartered by President Abraham Lincoln in 1861, Providence Hospital stands as the oldest continuously operating hospital in the Nation's Capital and a symbol of commitment to the healthcare needs of the metropolitan area. The 382-bed medical facility and 240-bed nursing and rehabilitation center fulfill the mission to the sick and the poor with joy, care, and respect, while at the same time embracing the best that medical science has to offer."[112]

to Dr. Robert Jacobson, a hematologist/oncologist who was interim chairman of medicine from 1988 to 1992,* Griffith held a senior faculty leadership retreat. "The emphasis at the end of the retreat was to focus all efforts to build up the cardiology, oncology, neurosciences, and surgical specialty services. No mention was made of primary care as a high priority." Soon afterwards, "all of this was ignored."[30]

Jacobson remembers that Father Leo O'Donovan, the recently installed university president, attended the retreat and "endorsed the aims of the faculty. He had a strong desire to build a first-rate medical center and commit resources to that endeavor. Yet, in my view, when the efforts turned to primary care and specialty services like cardiology withered, he was as frustrated as everyone else that the goals had not been achieved."[30] O'Donovan, a premedical student as an undergraduate,[28] later a theologian,[27] consistently favored the medical school,[77] unlike Timothy Healy, his predecessor at Georgetown, and Stephen Trachtenberg at George Washington.[15] Furthermore, O'Donovan believed that medical schools should be important features of Jesuit universities.[77]

Despite objections, Griffith proceeded with his reorientation of some parts of Georgetown clinical medicine toward primary care with the creation of the Community Health Network and the recruitment of Dr. John Eisenberg, one of the founders of the field of academic general internal medicine, as chairman of the department of medicine. Eisenberg, Griffith hoped, would develop strong academic programs in the administration and economics of health care.[11]

The clinical results were disappointing. In addition to not increasing referrals as much as hoped, the emphasis on primary care led to the departure of several of Georgetown's more eminent specialists.[11] The leaders were finding that the emphasis on primary care was not helping the troubled Georgetown University Hospital as much as predicted, a conclusion also being reached at other academic medical centers.[113]

Soon after acquiring the hospital and practice plan, MedStar closed the clinics.[73,77,79] "As for the leases, we ate them," said hospital president Joy Drass.[67] Most of the doctors in the practices "set up their own offices or took other jobs, though a few returned to teach at the main campus," according to Siwek.[79]

---

*Jacobson is now clinical research director of the Palm Beach Cancer Institute and director of its bone marrow/stem cell transplant program.

CHAPTER SEVEN

Georgetown University

Selling the Practice Plan

Georgetown developed the Faculty Physician Group (FPG), a consolidated practice plan for its full-time clinicians, in the early 1980s. Previously, the full-time faculty had been small, and most of the clinicians practiced privately. These volunteers, who were often graduates of the medical school or its training programs, admitted most of their patients to Georgetown University Hospital but saw their outpatients in private offices off the campus. A few worked as "geographical full-time" doctors, receiving some money from the medical school for teaching or administrative work and supplementing this with the proceeds from their practices.[1] Some described the hospital during these years as a "glorified community hospital" with a few strong programs.[2,3]

As part of his aim to develop a more research-based medical school at Georgetown, John Griffith, the executive vice president, increased the size of the full-time faculty. This led to the departure to other hospitals of many members of the voluntary faculty, whom the school did little to retain[3] and, in some cases, encouraged to leave.[4] In the department of surgery, for example, the chairman gave the best time in the operating rooms to the full-time faculty. Those voluntary surgeons who still worked at Georgetown found themselves having to operate at less desirable times.[5] "We were not practitioner-friendly," acknowledged one of the deans.[6]

Beginning in 1993, the medical center instituted an incentive plan to encourage the full-time clinicians to run busy, well-managed practices. One of the effects of this policy was to decrease the salaries of some of the clinicians by as much as 25 percent. Many of the less productive doctors left to work elsewhere or to take different jobs. Those who stayed tended to have the largest practices.[7]

By introducing the incentive scheme and by tightening operational practices, FPG began to generate a small surplus in spite of paying 5 percent of its gross revenue to the school of medicine, 1 percent to itself for infrastructure, and 1.5 percent to operate a group of satellite clinics the practice had developed.[3] Although several departments were still in deficit, the money received for teaching from the school of medicine and for doctors to perform services for the hospital enabled the plan as a whole to break even when MedStar bought the hospital in 2000.[8] Prior to these reforms, the plan had lost money.[9]

Although MedStar was initially hesitant about absorbing the practice plan,[3] the company soon came to believe that including the clinicians, particularly the "right physicians,"[10] in its operations was wise, if not essential.[6] "If we didn't have the docs," hospital president Joy Drass has said, referring to the full-time clinicians who accounted for at least 80 percent of the admissions,[10] "we couldn't have turned the hospital around. The doctors must be aligned with you for managed care, expense reduction, and incentives."[11]*

"When I was there, the practice plan wasn't controllable," said one of the pre-MedStar executives. "Everything had to be done in a collegial way. There's big frictional cost for collegiality."[12] "Such people need control because they're 'academic,'" one doctor heard a MedStar executive say. Accustomed to what MedStar saw as the easygoing life of the typical university physician, the clinicians needed to see more patients and work more efficiently than they had when Georgetown owned the group.

The company eventually came to feel so strongly about absorbing the practice plan because its executives kept insisting that "unless the doc-

---

*Few physicians in private practice, who at one time admitted many patients to the hospital, remained at Georgetown.

tors [came] in, the deal would be off." MedStar would not accept an arrangement as at George Washington in which full-time clinicians work in an independent corporation. They had to work for the company.[11,13-15] "MedStar perceived that the clinical faculty was the real strength of the medical school," Ken Bloem said. "That's what they were buying, more than the physical stuff."[16]

The university was in no position to oppose what MedStar insisted on. "We really had no choice," said Jack DeGioia.[17] Although the plan was not then losing money,[18] the university was concerned that it might in the future.* The clinical leaders, who had long operated independent of the university, "felt more comfortable with MedStar than with Georgetown," Bloem thought.[16]

When MedStar took it over, the Faculty Practice Group was renamed the Georgetown Practice Group (GPG).[7] Richard Goldberg, the current director, reports for this activity to the hospital president, Joy Drass. "It's not a true group practice," says Drass, "and it's unique."[11]

"Very Unpopular"

The takeover of the practice plan prescribed that most[20] of the clinicians providing clinical care and all their staff members become MedStar employees[11,21,22] at the same salaries they were earning at Georgetown.[23] After one year with their former Georgetown arrangements, each clinician would receive a twelve-month renewable term contract with MedStar. None would be tenured.[24,25] The company can discharge any of the doctors without cause 180 days after notifying them.[24] Physicians can terminate their employment agreement with ninety days' notice.[26]

"We were being sold but would still be university faculty," many of the doctors thought.[22]† "Teaching," one of the chairmen observed, "no longer bought university employment."[22] Financial support for clinical education was paid by the students' tuition. The funds flowed from the medical school to MedStar and, finally, "to us."[22]‡

*Some members of the faculty thought that the plan depended on a subsidy from the hospital in order not to lose money.[19]

†Until the physicians were actually transferred from university to MedStar employment, many in the clinical faculty believed or, perhaps more accurately, hoped that they could remain university employees.[22]

‡MedStar pays Georgetown for the clinical work performed by doctors employed by the university.[20]

Georgetown bought out the tenure of twenty-one members of the clinical faculty with tenure[3,21,23,27,28] by giving them, in a single payment, a sum that equaled one-and-a-half to two times their annual salary, which, in some cases, was significantly more than they were earning in clinical practice.[27] The buyout cost the university as much as $750,000 for some of the doctors.[3] Clinicians in the tenure track but without tenure received certain benefits as partial compensation for their losing the opportunity of ever becoming tenured at Georgetown.[20]

Georgetown had computed that buying the tenure would cost the university less, in the long run, than maintaining responsibility for paying the tenured faculty until they retired.* Although several members of the tenured clinical faculty opposed this change[30]—one chairman called it "very unpopular"[31]—only two refused the offer.[29] Those faculty members who had hoped or expected to gain tenure in the near future were disappointed, and some were angry.[25,27,30]

One who refused the buyout was the cardiothoracic surgeon Nevin Katz, a tenured professor of surgery and chief of adult cardiac surgery at Georgetown when MedStar bought the hospital and practice plan. "I learned that Georgetown would no longer honor tenure for the clinical faculty," Katz said. "MedStar had made it clear that their surgeons from the Washington Hospital Center would take over and that I wouldn't be welcome as part of their program."[32] Katz unsuccessfully challenged the university for revoking his tenure and, upon suing to obtain a one-year notice before being discharged, again unsuccessfully,[33] moved to George Washington.

Michael Pentecost, the chairman of radiology, was the other. Rejecting the buyout meant that he lost his university job on July 1, 2000. Like Nevin Katz, he unsuccessfully sued to recover his tenure. The university claimed that it was in "financial exigency" and could accordingly terminate tenure when required. The basis for Pentecost's case was, according to him, "a straight issue of academic freedom."[34] He held that the tenured clinical faculty should have the option to accept or reject the offer without losing their university jobs as is usual at other universities that offer to buy out tenure electively to decrease the size of the senior faculty.[35]†

---

*John DeGioia, then the university senior vice president, later the president, met with each member of the tenured faculty to develop the settlements.[29]

†In 2005, Pentecost left Georgetown and MedStar to become director of the Institute for Health Policy in Radiology of the American College of Radiology and chief of radiology at the Mid-Atlantic Permanente Medical Group at Kaiser Permanente in Rockville, Maryland.[34]

DeGioia and the Georgetown lawyers decided to deal with other disaffected faculty members as gently as possible—although Nevin Katz and Michael Pentecost would deny that that was how they were treated and handle lawsuits as they came up.

Since the clinicians could expect to receive no support from the university after MedStar took over, most joined the company except for those in the Lombardi Cancer Center and a few others, whom the university retained.[11] The clinicians had been given no choice. They either had to join MedStar or leave.[36] Among those who stayed, many remained worried about their future employment.[22]

Three hundred and fifty-four of the approximately four hundred members of the clinical faculty accepted the MedStar offer of employment in July 2000.[26] Clinicians who did not favor the new arrangement or distrusted MedStar went into private practice or took other jobs.[22,23,27,30,37] Members of the nonprofessional staff who did not want to work for MedStar had to leave; a few found jobs at the university.[7]

What the university and MedStar had worked out displeased many of the clinicians. They remember the process as a "contentious issue," that the university had "abrogated its responsibilities to the faculty." "Some of us should have been allowed to remain [as university employees]," said one of the senior clinicians.[30]

Clinical faculty who went to MedStar now receive one paycheck, and it is from MedStar, no longer from the university. Benefits changed so much that some faculty members resigned or retired on this issue alone.[22,23,34,38-43]

- *Pension.* Compared with Georgetown, MedStar contributes significantly less to the pension plan, does not allow immediate vesting, and prohibits employees from controlling how their retirement money is invested.
- *Tuition.* Georgetown clinicians hired by MedStar after 2000 lost the benefit of free tuition for them and their dependents to attend Georgetown or reduced tuition at other colleges and universities. Faculty and staff who had been eligible for the tuition benefit and had been Georgetown employees for at least three years before 2000 would continue to receive this benefit until 2008.[20] The university pays the cost for this subsidy.

- *Tenure.* No clinicians employed by MedStar have university tenure. "As Georgetown no longer retains those who work primarily in clinical care," a university official explains, "Georgetown no longer employs or tenures 'clinicians.' "[44]
- *The university grievance mechanism* is no longer available to MedStar-employed clinical faculty.
- *Status* as employees of the university. Clinical faculty who became MedStar employees lost this.

Parking also became an issue.[14] MedStar wanted more spaces for what, it hoped, would be more patients. Since community opposition prevented building more parking facilities, some of the university faculty were forced to park in a less convenient lot.[45]

"It was a very difficult time," one of the chairmen remembered,[22] "a PR nightmare" said another,[29] "not a popular switch, no one had a choice," said a third.[39] Richard Goldberg added, "The divorce from the university was much worse than the marriage with MedStar."[3] Dr. Steven Epstein, Goldberg's successor as chairman of psychiatry, said, "It was a forced marriage, but it's worked out much better than anyone imagined."[22]

Those members of the clinical faculty whose principal work was research, education, or administration could remain employees of the university. They constituted from about 20 percent in those departments with research programs to none in departments with primarily clinical activities. MedStar insisted that all permanent chairmen of the clinical departments be MedStar employees.* Basic scientists, including those in the clinical departments, remained employees of the university.[21]

"Sam Took a Terrible Beating"

The satisfactory completion of these delicate negotiations depended greatly on the skills of Sam Wiesel. "Sam was the right man at the right time," says Richard Goldberg, who believes that, without Wiesel, "there'd be no medical enterprise at Georgetown."[3] Others agree.[21]

Seen by some as having "an idiosyncratic view of the world, strongly opinionated, even autocratic,"[46] Wiesel had more than his share of problems, one of which was encouraging unproductive full-time clinicians to

*See below.

leave.[47] He also tried to limit the income of faculty who lost their grants or whose practices could not support their salaries and offered to buy out the contracts of some whom he thought unproductive.[9,48] Accordingly, some of the aggrieved called the orthopedist "an amputation surgeon"[49] because "he had so much bad news to bring to the clinicians."[50]

"The basic scientists faulted Sam for not being a sophisticated investigator," said Michael Kelly, the university vice president.[50] This was a problem recognized by many others[9,13,19,22,24,29,31,46,48,51-55] and not denied by Wiesel.[28] "Sam was looking after the clinical docs, not us," complained one of the basic science chairmen.

Some criticized the university for appointing Wiesel to the position of executive vice president and executive dean, for which they thought he had little preparation or appropriate experience.[19] Others accused him of conflict of interest because he was negotiating with MedStar while knowing that he would eventually become a MedStar employee.[19]* Disgruntled faculty even tried, unsuccessfully, to have him removed from his job in 2000.[48,56]

"Sam took a terrible beating," remembers Kelly. "He had a dreadful job to do."[50] One of the administrators added, "Sam must have very tough skin."[9]

Despite the turmoil, however, medicine at Georgetown survived. Some thought that "the medical school and hospital would have closed if Sam hadn't been able to work it out with MedStar and Jack [DeGioia, the university president]," psychiatrist Steven Epstein explains. "Of course, recognizing that George Washington was having similar problems helped our morale."[22] Jay Siwek from family medicine adds, "Sam brought us together."[42]

As for Wiesel's immediate future at Georgetown after MedStar took over, he continued to direct the medical center† to which was added the job of chief medical officer of the hospital, but he had lost authority for the hospital and practice plan to MedStar. By 2002, with the medical center[51] and MedStar desiring new leadership and encouraged by Joy Drass,[57] Wiesel relinquished the positions he still had and returned to directing the department of orthopedic surgery on a full-time basis. Former psychiatry chairman Richard Goldberg succeeded him as chief medical officer of the hospital.[7]

---

*The university formed an interim structure, the Committee for Transitional Administration of the Medical Center, to work with Wiesel and "manage any apparent or actual conflicts of interest."[20]

†The university prefers to use the phrase "medical center" where many, including the author, would say "medical school." I have adopted Georgetown's preference.

Joy Drass remembers hearing that the doctors blamed Georgetown rather than MedStar for forcing their separation.[11] "They've become much happier since the hospital has become such a better place to work, and we're not afraid to make decisions," says the senior MedStar executive on the Georgetown campus.[11] Stephen Evans, the chairman of surgery since 2002, agrees. "The hospital knows that its success depends primarily on its doctors. The practice plan supports the hospital."[58] Neurology chairman Edward Healton says, "MedStar gives us excellent support. Being a MedStar employee is not a problem."[59]

Not all agree, however, that selling the practice plan was wise. The clinical chairmen were not pleased by the loss of some of their administrative and financial powers to MedStar.[60] Dr. Marc Lippman, director of the Lombardi Cancer Center from 1988 to 2001, believes that Georgetown did not need to sell the practice plan and considers doing so "a bigger mistake than selling the hospital." He regrets particularly that the school will lose potential philanthropy that full-time doctors can develop from grateful patients.[61]*

Michael Pentecost also thought selling the practice plan "very disquieting. How can Georgetown now recruit top-notch academics?"[34]—a question that continues to be asked by many of his former colleagues. "They panicked," Lippman added, "and decided that Georgetown simply didn't belong in the medical industry."[61] And that is what happened. After MedStar had absorbed the hospital and the practice plan, Georgetown, the school from which Joy Drass had graduated, was, as she explained, "no longer in the clinical business."[11]

Lombardi Cancer Center

The clinical unit that seems to have best survived the turmoil at Georgetown is the Lombardi Comprehensive Cancer Center.[51,62] The unit is named for Vince Lombardi, the legendary head coach of the Washington Redskins who died of widespread colon cancer in September 1970.[51] Georgetown doctors had treated Lombardi for what they soon recognized to be an un-

---

*A university official adds: "Although there was a brief period of time (in 2005) when GUH [Georgetown University] and GUMC [Georgetown University Medical Center] did not partner for fundraising and share prospect lists, the development partnership is strong and was made stronger in 2005 by a joint agreement that recognizes that the philanthropic fortunes of the two institutions are inextricably linked and provides a collaborative framework for pooling resources and pursuing projects and objectives of common interest."[44]

treatable lesion. "He was heroic about his illness and his impending death," remembered Dr. John Potter, the oncology surgeon who had participated in his care. "We decided to name our cancer center for him."[60] Georgetown's connection with the team had included providing the use of one of the university's fields for the Redskins to practice.[64]

In 1973 the center applied for a core and construction grant from the National Institutes of Health (NIH), which was approved for $275,000, "then a lot of money," Potter, the director of the center at the time, remembers.[63] In 1974, the NIH designated the unit as its seventeenth comprehensive cancer center and two years later awarded $4 million for a building to house the center, which would open in 1982. The lawyer Edward Bennett Williams then chaired an advisory committee that raised additional funds. The National Football League gave a one-time gift of $1 million in Lombardi's name. By 1986, Georgetown's cancer center employed eighty-five senior professional staff with M.D. or Ph.D. degrees, had an endowment of $2.4 million, and brought in $5.2 million per year in patient fees and research grants.*

Marc Lippman, who succeeded Potter as director of the Lombardi, came from the National Cancer Institute (NCI), where he had been head of the medical breast cancer section since 1976.† Bringing thirty of his NCI colleagues with him into a building that was three-quarters empty,[51] Lippman greatly expanded what became the Washington area's premier nongovernmental center for the care of patients with cancer. He administered the basic science research through the cancer center and the clinical care through the relevant departments.[51] Under Lippman, Lombardi grew into a leader in clinical and basic research in cancer as its share of patients in the market increased from 4 to 20 percent while the hospital's share was stagnating at about 4 percent.[61] Despite its success, however, the hospital limited how large Lombardi could become.[65]

By the time he left in 2001 to become chairman of the department of medicine at the University of Michigan, Lippman had become disillusioned with medicine at Georgetown. With most faculty recruitment becoming frozen in the school, "I didn't want to tear down what my prede-

---

*Potter by now "had had enough of administration," so he resigned as the director but continued working at Georgetown as chief of surgical oncology. In 2000 he closed his practice and became director of the United States Military Cancer Institute of the Uniformed Services University of the Health Sciences in Bethesda, Maryland.[63]

†"Marc's recruitment was my last official act," remembers former dean Milton Corn, "and one that I'm particularly proud of."[62]

cessors and I had built," he said.* "No one saw the troubles that were coming, and no one seemed aware of what needed to be fixed."[61] Lippman feared that the Lombardi might lose its cancer center grant after MedStar took over.[51]†

Dr. Kevin Cullen, whom Lippman had brought from the NIH, succeeded him as acting director. Cullen established the Betty Lou Ourisman Breast Cancer Clinic, recruited fifteen new faculty members, and prepared Lombardi for the successful renewal in 2003 of its designation as a Comprehensive Cancer Center of the NCI.‡ In 2004, Cullen became director of the cancer center at the University of Maryland.

Cullen's successor at Georgetown departed after a few years.§ The Lombardi was led by an acting director until the appointment of Dr. Louis Wiener, chairman of the department of medical oncology at the Fox Chase Cancer Center in Philadelphia, who became director in January 2008.

In addition to Marc Lippman, other leaders with strong investigative programs like Robert Martuza, the chairman of neurosurgery,[54] and Jeffrey Cossman, the chairman of pathology, also left at about the same time.[67]**

Education

"The students and house staff didn't notice a thing when MedStar took over. The conversion was seamless," said Richard Goldberg, the chief medical officer of the hospital and vice president for medical affairs at Georgetown.[3] Dean for medical education Ray Mitchell comments:[68]

> Our match days have been progressively more successful in the last five years. In 2006, nearly 40 percent of Georgetown students matched into top-ranked pro-

* "Most of the NCI scientists Lippman had recruited chose to stay at Georgetown rather than follow Lippman to Michigan," a medical center official responds.[44]

† In May 2007, Lippman left Michigan to become chairman of the department of medicine at the University of Miami.

‡ According to executive vice president Bondurant, "The center is stronger financially than it has been in the past. Research dollars have increased steadily—from $11.8 million in sponsored research funding during 1993 to $44.6 million in 2006—and patient care responsibilities are also larger."[66]

§ Dr. Richard Pestell, Lippman's successor, now works at the Jefferson Medical College in Philadelphia. Dr. Pestell declined to be interviewed for this book.

** Cossman remembers the period from 1990 to 1995 as a time when medical research at Georgetown flourished. He recruited more than fifteen new faculty members to his department, and by the time he left, he and his colleagues held forty grants, including some from the NIH. "The department had only one non-NIH grant when I started as chairman in 1989," he remembers. "What's happened since then is a terrible shame."[67] Cossman is now chief scientific officer of the Critical Path Institute, Rockville, Maryland.

grams in highly competitive medical specialties this year, including those at Harvard University, Duke University Medical Center, Mayo Graduate School of Medicine, and Columbia University Medical Center.

The School of Medicine has been in *U.S. News & World Report*'s top fifty listing of medical schools every year except one (2003) since the transaction, and its ranking has remained strong.

Applications are up by 17 percent this year (compared to a national average of 8 percent) to the School of Medicine—more than 10,600 applications for 191 spots.

In 2005, the Liaison Committee on Medical Education (LCME) reaccredited the school until 2010.

Opinions differ about whether the quality of clinical education for the medical students and trainees has suffered or improved when compared with pre-MedStar days.[3,6,36,39,49,60,64] Those who say that the education programs, especially for students, are worse ascribe the problem to MedStar's incentive system, which requires the clinicians to spend more time practicing, thereby reducing their availability for teaching. However, the increased inpatient census at the Georgetown hospital since MedStar made its changes means more patients for students to work with.

The medical school paid MedStar and the hospital $9 million during 2006–7 for teaching performed by the MedStar-employed clinical faculty. This includes education for the medical students in their third and fourth clinical years and a significant portion of their teaching during the first and second years. The school pays $3.5 million to the basic science departments for the teaching performed by the university faculty during the preclinical years.[69]

James Spies, the radiology chairman, believes that the residency programs have significantly improved. "They're better because they're more rigorous. The programs and the house staff have to obey the rules [about working hours, for example], and we have internal reviews now."[70]

The merger, however, has caused problems for some departments in training their residents and fellows. The department of ophthalmology, for example, had to close its subspecialty fellowship program, the former chairman Dr. Howard Cupples explained, because, when the merger occurred, the university took the surplus his department had saved.[38]* "Too expen-

---

*The university also prevented the department of pediatrics from spending money it had saved. "The university and I got into quite a fight over this," Dr. Owen Rennert, chairman of the department

sive," Cupples was told when he asked MedStar executives to pay for the fellows.[38]*

The department of ophthalmology remains small, with only two full-time members. Seven members of the clinical faculty, who help teach the students and residents, "see patients in leased space in the Pasquerilla building on campus and in their offices elsewhere. Though we're not currently a high priority for the hospital, we consistently receive the resources and support that we need from the administration," explains Dr. Jay Lustbader, Cupples's successor as chairman in 2005.[40]†

With MedStar now owning both the Washington Hospital Center and the Georgetown University Hospital, affiliations between them have grown. Increasing numbers of students and trainees from each hospital receive part of their education at the other. One result of this has been to diminish the number training at Fairfax Hospital in Northern Virginia. With Georgetown now allied with MedStar and no longer as dependent on Fairfax for training opportunities, Fairfax turned to George Washington to replace some of the agreements formerly made with Georgetown.[71]

Chairmen of Clinical Departments

Four doctors, as permanent or interim, have chaired the department of medicine‡ since Dr. John Eisenberg was recruited from the University of Pennsylvania in 1992.§ Under Eisenberg, according to Karen Campbell, his administrator, division chiefs were recruited, funding for research grants tripled, a surplus was generated each year that he was chairman, and the house staff program became more competitive. Before Eisenberg, the Georgetown medical internship program did not fill its annual quota.[24]

---

from 1988 to 1998, said.[55] Rennert, a strongly academic pediatrician, is remembered by one of his colleagues as a man whose motto was "do good more than do well."[2] He is now scientific director of the National Institute of Child Health and Human Development of the NIH.

  *Fellowships, the programs that train subspecialists after finishing their residencies, are supported by departments and divisions in medical schools, at least partly, and not by hospitals in many academic medical centers.

  †Lustbader, like many of the current chairmen, was appointed without a national search.[40]

  ‡For a history of the department of medicine from the founding to 1981, see "Upward Journey. The Story of Internal Medicine at Georgetown, 1851–1981" by Dr. John Stapleton.[72]

  §Stuart Bondurant, a former chairman of medicine himself, remembers an article showing that "the half life of chairs of departments of medicine nationally was less than four years. With four chairs in fourteen years, GU's [Georgetown University] average is very close to that."[66]

Despite these accomplishments, several members of the faculty, displeased by his leadership, petitioned John Griffith, who had hired him, not to continue his chairmanship. Accordingly, Griffith told Eisenberg that he would not renew his contract when it ended five years after he arrived at Georgetown.[24] "Personal agendas forced him out," in Campbell's opinion.[24] Upon leaving the university, Eisenberg became director of the federal Agency for Healthcare Research and Quality.*

Eisenberg was succeeded by the vice chairman, immunologist Dr. Paul Katz,[24] a second-generation alumnus of the Georgetown medical school. Later, Wiesel appointed Katz chief operating officer of the hospital, a position that increasingly took more of his time at the expense of the chairmanship. Katz often had to decide whether a particular professional or financial decision better suited the hospital or the department. In the conflict of interest that holding these two jobs simultaneously inevitably produced, "medicine usually lost," according to Campbell. "The faculty was beginning to feel abandoned and believed that there was no one to advocate for the department."[24]

With the arrival of MedStar, Katz returned to the medicine chairmanship full-time. His job, however was no longer the same as it had been. For example, he learned after the fact—"just to let you know," as Katz remembers being informed[29]—that MedStar had assigned one of its cardiologists from the Washington Hospital Center to run the service in Katz's department at Georgetown.

Katz became frustrated by MedStar's assumption of authority for the department's clinical responsibilities. Unable to achieve authority at least equal to what he had formerly exercised as chief operating officer, powerless to affect what he saw as MedStar's degrading of the academic mission, and disappointed that his talents were not being better recognized at Georgetown, Katz soon left.[29]† Joy Drass, the hospital president who had been Katz's classmate in medical school,[74] did not object.[51] It was thought, by a Katz supporter, that the reason she did not retain him in December

---

*Eisenberg died of a brain tumor on March 10, 2002, at the age of fifty-five.[73] *Disclosure:* The author, a friend of John Eisenberg, taught him when he was a resident at the Hospital of the University of Pennsylvania and worked with him there for several years when they were both members of the medical faculty at the University of Pennsylvania.

†Upon leaving Georgetown, Katz became senior vice president and chief medical officer of the Mount Sinai Medical Center and Miami Heart Institute in Miami Beach, Florida, and professor of medicine at the University of Miami School of Medicine.

2000 was because Drass and the new MedStar executives felt threatened by Katz's comprehensive knowledge of Georgetown medicine.[24] What action Sam Wiesel, the medical center's executive vice president and executive dean at the time, took with relation to Katz's leaving is not known.*

Dr. Richard Waldhorn, a Georgetown pulmonologist, succeeded Katz as interim chairman for one year and then became permanent chairman in 2002. By 2004, however, Waldhorn explains, "I had done each job in the department and was weary of administration. I'd run out of things to do, and it was no longer fun."[25] Waldhorn, who left after having been chairman for only two years, thereby became the second consecutive chairman of medicine to depart Georgetown after MedStar took over.† Dr. Joseph Verbalis, who came to Georgetown in 1995 as chief of endocrinology, has been interim chairman since then.[74]

Neurology also suffered from rotating chairs. Dr. Kimford Meador had been recruited to Georgetown from the Medical College of Georgia to become chairman in 2002. Unlike many senior appointments at the time, Meador's selection was the result of a national search because of Georgetown's and MedStar's interest in developing the neurosciences. "I was enthusiastic," he remembers. "Neurosurgery at Georgetown was strong, and working with the National Rehabilitation Hospital [owned by MedStar on the Washington Hospital Center campus] and other hospitals in the MedStar system offered great opportunities."[57]

Meador's passion for his job was short lived. The cause, he said, was "MedStar, not the medical school,"[57] an attribution that MedStar emphatically denies.[26] Soon after Meador arrived, he asserts, the hospital reduced the department's financial support below the amount that Meador had negotiated when accepting the job. Meador and his colleagues were particularly annoyed when MedStar started a program in epilepsy surgery to be staffed by private practitioners at the Washington Hospital Center. This would directly compete with the program Meador, a specialist in the field, was trying to develop at Georgetown University Hospital. Meador stated that "this action undermined the development of the Georgetown neurol-

*When asked about this episode, Wiesel replied that confidentiality arrangements prevented his commenting.[75]

†Waldhorn, a pulmonologist who had been at Georgetown for twenty-eight years, is now senior investigator at the Center for Biosecurity in Baltimore and distinguished scholar at the University of Pittsburgh. He continues to live in a Washington suburb.

ogy program and demonstrated that there was no coordination of programs across the MedStar system."[57]

Finally, Meador says, "Joy [Drass] delayed negotiated funding [Drass denies this[76]] and reduced the amount of support that was promised to recruit new faculty in neurology." Meador communicated his problems to the central MedStar office and expressed his willingness to meet with senior officers. MedStar never asked him to attend a meeting to discuss his concerns, he says. Making himself available for a new job, Meador accepted an endowed chair in neurology at the University of Florida in Gainesville and left in 2004, only two years after coming to Georgetown.[57]

One of the more controversial results of the merger is MedStar's insistence that every chairman of a clinical department must be a MedStar employee. All but one of the permanent clinical chairmen switched to MedStar[25] after receiving the lump sum that came with the university's buying out the tenure of those who had it. Interim medicine chairman Joseph Verbalis,[74] among others,[25] sees this policy as flawed because it will inhibit the recruitment of chairmen with strong academic, as opposed to strictly clinical or administrative, interests. Under this rule, Verbalis is ineligible to become the permanent chairman of medicine unless he transfers his employment from Georgetown to MedStar.

In Verbalis's department, about 17 percent of the full-time faculty, including the interim chairman, remain university employees. These include faculty members who primarily educate and investigate and spend less than about 50 percent of their time in clinical work and all those with research degrees such as the Ph.D.[74]

Many wonder if Georgetown and MedStar will be able to recruit the type of candidate who fills this position at leading medical schools. Medicine chairmen traditionally have strong academic records and have carried out important basic or clinical research. Most come from directorships of specialty divisions and have learned how to recruit faculty, administer complex academic projects, handle budgets, and relate constructively to hospital executives and their medical school colleagues. They will need money and space to recruit faculty for weak divisions. Many potential chairmen from other institutions, like Verbalis at Georgetown, may look suspiciously at becoming employees of MedStar and not the university and reporting for clinical activities to a CEO and not a dean.

Creation of co-chairs has been proposed to deal with the clinical/

research impasse. The academic chair would be employed by Georgetown and the clinical chair by MedStar. Theoretically, the dean could hire and relieve the academic chair, as could MedStar for the clinical chair. Radiology briefly had two chairs.[6] Michael Pentecost had previously been the sole chairman, but his orientation toward academic duties led to the separation of these responsibilities. Drass then assigned them to a colleague who would concentrate on operations. Anesthesia briefly had dual chairmen, but the only department now so structured is pathology.* "No one liked or wanted the system [of co-chairs]," said Verbalis.[74] Others agree[6,35] and emphasize the difficulty convincing suitable candidates from other schools to come to Georgetown to lead departments with dual chairs.[35]

The sale of the practice plan to MedStar affects some Georgetown departments more than others. For departments such as orthopedic surgery, with a predominately clinical mission, the merger has presented few problems, and of course, the basic science departments are not involved since they remain in the medical center. The greatest difficulties arise in those clinical departments, such as medicine and pediatrics, with larger research components in addition to clinical programs.

The permanent clinical chairmen, whom MedStar insists it must employ,[25,74] now relate to four administrative centers: the hospital president for clinical issues, the dean for medical education for medical student teaching, the director of the biomedical graduate research organization (BGRO)† for research, and the executive vice president for senior administrative matters. Some find that this change adds additional administrative burdens in the management of academic departments.[21] Others see it as less of a problem.[59]

Serving more than one master can be complicated,[38] "taking much en-

---

*Dr. Richard Schlegel, a university employee, is the academic chairman of the department of pathology and responsible for teaching the medical students and for research, in his case viral oncology. One member of the department on the university payroll receives some money from MedStar for teaching the students in their clinical years. With the transfer of clinical oncology to MedStar, the departure of investigators, and the freeze on recruiting, Schlegel's laboratory is the only one left in the department, and he is the only remaining tenured faculty member. Three assistant professors on three-year contracts work with him. According to the recently instituted reorganization of the medical center, pathology is administratively assigned to the Lombardi Comprehensive Cancer Center and the department's paperwork is handled by the Lombardi administrator.[77]

Dr. Norio Azumi, the clinical chairman, directs clinical pathology in the hospital. He is employed by MedStar and reports to Joy Drass, the hospital president.

†See below.

ergy, which is not productive and produces bad feelings," says former medicine chairman Richard Waldhorn. "The system makes it difficult to keep our department's tripartite mission [clinical care, teaching, and research] together. It's not worth it for what was accomplished and is not universally endorsed as a great plan."[25]

Powers of the Dean

It is the impression of several members of the senior faculty that the hospital president now influences the appointment and discharge of the clinical chairs more directly than is usual at most academic medical centers.[7,74,78] Though most chairmen of the clinical departments and division chiefs continued in their roles when MedStar took over, when an opening develops, MedStar has an important role in deciding who gets the job.

The clinical chairmen recommend the doctors' salaries, which must be approved by two hospital officials, Richard Goldberg, the chief medical officer, and Joy Drass, the president.[7,60] Thus, as MedStar employees, the clinicians' jobs depend primarily, as Stuart Bondurant says, "on satisfying the goals of the company, which include the support of teaching and research as expressed by covering the deficit of the MedStar Research Institute,"[79]* and no longer the dean. According to some, this causes problems for the dean when he wants to convince members of the clinical faculty to conduct clinical research since their jobs depend primarily upon doing what counts most to MedStar: running active, successful practices.† Consequently, recruiting clinical investigators has become increasingly difficult.

Since the dean no longer directs the practice plan, he cannot tax the financially successful clinical departments to support clinical and basic science departments needing development or operating funds. Yet the dean has to pay MedStar for teaching the medical students by the clinicians who were formerly part of the university system.[25] With the dean receiving no direct support from the hospital, it follows that the medical center remains in financial difficulty.‡ Because the clinicians are not specifically paid for it,

*See chapter 9.
†According to Bondurant, "This is a widely held opinion, but this judgment is not buttressed by any data."[66]
‡"The medical center does receive substantial indirect support from the hospital in many forms: basic science teaching by clinical faculty, as an example," Bondurant adds.[79]

one former clinical chairman found it necessary "to beg the clinical faculty to teach the house staff"[25] as do the basic science chairmen who need clinicians to teach the medical students part of their courses.[64]

The principal criticism leveled at MedStar from many members of the faculty is that the company is only interested in "dollars and practice, not in academics." Interim executive vice president Stuart Bondurant, who was dean of the University of North Carolina School of Medicine in Chapel Hill from 1979 to 1994, holds that MedStar's control of the practice plan "means less now than it did at the beginning. The students and residents can't tell the difference. Our students matched better than ever, and the LCME [Liaison Committee on Medical Education] gave us full accreditation."[46]

Combining Clinical Departments and Training Programs

Since MedStar bought the Georgetown University Hospital and its Faculty Practice Group in July 2000, leaders at MedStar have been studying which professional functions can be combined at the Washington Hospital Center and the Georgetown hospital.* As of the summer of 2006, the only merged department was emergency medicine, which had been consolidated under a single chairman based at the Hospital Center. Dr. Mark Smith knows the local scene well. Having trained at George Washington and Georgetown, Smith directed GW's department from 1985 to 1995, when he and several of his colleagues moved to the Washington Hospital Center with Smith as chairman of the service.

When MedStar acquired Georgetown, Joy Drass asked that the Washington Hospital Center emergency physician group provide physician leadership and direction at Georgetown. The university then appointed Smith professor of emergency medicine and confirmed MedStar's selection of him as chairman of the department at the medical school. In addition, the MedStar Emergency Physician group directed by Smith provides emergency services at MedStar's Franklin Square Hospital—which, Smith says, has the busiest emergency department in Maryland—and Union Memorial Hospital, both of which are in Baltimore.[81]

The division of cardiology has recently been consolidated. Based at the

---

*The executives at other merged teaching hospitals have also tried to combine clinical programs, usually unsuccessfully, and training programs, more successfully.[80]

Hospital Center, where most of the program is conducted, Leslie Miller also directs the much-reduced cardiology activities at the Georgetown hospital.[82]

MedStar and Georgetown asked Dr. Leonard Wartofsky, the chairman of medicine at the Washington Hospital Center, to consider becoming the first chairman of a combined department of medicine after Richard Waldhorn left as chairman in 2004.[83] The initiative failed. Wartofsky was disappointed that Joy Drass had taken a leading role in restructuring the compensation scheme in the gastrointestinal (GI) division, thereby changing the traditional reporting relationship between that division and the department. "That was the line in the sand," said Wartofsky. "I wanted to demonstrate that I had a charter to build the department and weakening the link between the GI division and the department killed that possibility."[83]

Drass explains that she did not change the reporting structure in the gastroenterology division. "I forced a new compensation plan in GI to replace what was a disincentive with incentives to practice more successfully," a technique MedStar is applying to the clinicians in all the clinical units.[84] "All section chiefs [continue to] report to their chair for clinical matters, and the chairs report to the medical director Rich Goldberg for clinical practice."[85]

Several residencies and fellowships—anesthesiology, cardiology, dermatology, emergency medicine, endocrinology, ophthalmology, otorhinolaryngology (ENT), psychosomatic medicine, urology, vascular and interventional radiology, transplant surgery, and vascular surgery—have been integrated. An applicant for one of these residencies or fellowships applies to the combined Georgetown–Washington Hospital Center program and not to separate programs at the two hospitals.[82] The trainees in those programs who have not been integrated but are affiliated may work at the other hospital for part of their experience.

Many of the programs at the Hospital Center have adopted the Georgetown name. For example, the department of medicine at the Hospital Center now calls its medical internship and residency program "Georgetown University Hospital/Washington Hospital Center Internal Medicine."[83,86]* The Georgetown connection has increased the competitive character of the Hospital Center program. Formerly, the Hospital Center had difficulty re-

---

*Georgetown has 105 medical residents, the Washington Hospital Center 71.[83]

cruiting well-qualified U.S. medical graduates into its categorical three-year program. "This is changing," said Wartofsky. "We are getting competitive American applicants and the best international graduates. The preliminary [the one-year program for graduates planning to specialize in fields other than internal medicine] has become very popular."[83]

Dr. Janis Orlowski, chief medical officer at the Washington Hospital Center,* says that discussions are continuing about whether such major departments as medicine or surgery might merge, but so far none has amalgamated. "The doctors aren't ready for it yet," she believes.[82] One clinical department that is unlikely ever to merge is obstetrics and gynecology. The strictures of the Catholic Church on abortion and related issues that apply at the Georgetown hospital are not acceptable to the Washington Hospital Center's physicians and administrators.[82]†

Many members of the clinical faculty are feeling better about the merger than they did when it started. "We're coming together as a system," says Edward Healton, the chairman of neurology, but he cautions that "looking backward is more destructive than looking forward."[59] Mark Smith adds, "Most of the squabbling has gone. The merger's working great."[81]

---

*Orlowski reports to Dr. William Thomas, MedStar's executive vice president for medical affairs, whose office is at the corporate headquarters in Columbia, Maryland, and to the president of the Washington Hospital Center.

†In other respects, however, MedStar has had little difficulty working with the Catholic nature of Georgetown. "We had the experience of previously working with Good Sam [Good Samaritan Hospital, the Catholic hospital in Baltimore]," said MedStar CEO John McDaniel.[87]

CHAPTER EIGHT

Georgetown University and Its Medical School

History*

Georgetown University, founded in 1789 and opened in January 1792, reflected the vision of John Carroll,[2]† "an American-born, European-educated Jesuit priest who returned to the United States in 1773 with the goal of securing the future of American Catholicism through education—in particular, through the establishment of a preeminent Catholic place of higher learning." Carroll insisted that the college "be opened to students of every religious profession," and nearly one-fifth of its students during the first ten years were Protestants. "Religious pluralism characterized Georgetown's student population."[3]

The medical school began when four local physicians, a Roman Catholic, an Episcopalian, a Methodist, and a Jew, successfully petitioned Georgetown College to form a Medical Department in 1849. The doctors would

---

*Much of this history has been adapted from the excellent chapter on the medical school by Dr. Milton Corn in the book *Georgetown at Two Hundred*, edited by William C. McFadden, S.J.[1]

† As described on the university's Web site.

bear responsibility for all expenses and were expected to pay back any loans they might receive from the college. As Milton Corn writes: "It was location, the prestige of the college, and above all, the school's power to award degrees, rather than the Catholic nature of Georgetown which attracted the attention of the founding physicians."[4]

The school opened in rented space on F Street near the corner of Twelfth Street, NW. The first class of eight students entered in 1850, and three graduated with M.D. degrees one year later. Dr. John Stapleton, the department of medicine's historian, described Georgetown's early years as "truly a struggle. Conducted autonomously by seven practicing physicians who taught everything, housed in sparse quarters, and lacking a hospital, the school offered lectures at night that led to a degree after two years. Admission requirements were minimal. Most students had not attended college. Although the school existed in the nation's capital, Washington was largely a provincial southern town, not yet a leading city."[5]

In 1886 the school moved into its own building on H Street between Ninth and Tenth streets. From 1870 to 1900 a maximum of thirty students graduated each year. In 1878, the course was extended from two to three years and in 1893 to four years, each of seven months' duration, and all-day attendance was required starting in 1895.

In his famous report of 1910, Abraham Flexner called Georgetown's medical school "a university department in name only." Neither Georgetown's or George Washington's schools, Flexner wrote, are "now equal to the task of training physicians of the modern type."[6]

Responding to Flexner, Georgetown organized the school into formal departments, increased the size of the faculty, most of whom continued to support themselves in private practice, and made all its basic science faculty full-time. By 1929, the size of the classes had grown to eighty and the faculty to 141. Not until 1938, however, was a bachelor's degree required for matriculation.

From its founding, the school had functioned under the control of its faculty and autonomous of the university. The assignment of a university official to act as regent of the medical school in the mid-1920s began the process of making the school part of the university functionally as well as nominally.

In 1930, the medical school moved to the university campus upon the construction of a building that would gradually become the hub of its current medical center (it is still in use today). The size of the classes would grow to its current number of about 190, making Georgetown one of the country's largest private medical schools* and among those that would charge the highest tuitions. It was not until 1947 that the school began admitting women as regular students in the first year class. The first African American students enrolled in 1960 and graduated in 1964.[8]

The school taught clinical medicine at several small hospitals in Washington throughout most of the nineteenth century. In 1898, the university provided space on its campus for a university hospital of 33 beds that gradually grew to 293 beds until, in 1947, the core of the current Georgetown University Hospital opened adjacent to the medical school with 407 beds.

Restructuring the Medical Center

Since 2000, the school has had to solve its financial and organizational problems without the participation of the hospital and practice plan, which it no longer controls. Acting with the support of the board of directors and the president of the university,[9] Stuart Bondurant took strong and, in many cases, unpopular measures to reduce the continuing losses in the medical school of $16.9 million (accrual basis)† in 2005–6, though 30 percent less than in 2003–4. Since the sale of the clinical enterprise to MedStar, the medical school has received no funds from the practice plan[11] or the hospital[12] to support research activities, aid on which the school had previously depended.[13]

Whether or not the hospital comes to the rescue, "we must tighten up management in the basic sciences," Bondurant explains. "Many operate too much in silos, solely within their own groups, the chairmen using their departments as fiefdoms and preventing interdepartmental research which we must encourage."[14] Bondurant wants to establish at Georgetown the collaborative environment he admired when dean of the medical school at the University of North Carolina (UNC).[14]

Such dreams notwithstanding, Bondurant has had to develop plans that would secure solvency for the medical center, and, he said, "pass the prudent man test" by:[14]

---

*For the class of 2010, Georgetown received about 8,800 applicants. Three hundred eighty-three were offered positions, and 191 matriculated.[7]

†The cash deficit during 2006 was between $8 and $10 million.[10]

- Restructuring the central administration of the school
- Completing a reorganization of the basic science departments
- Meeting the budget for 2006–7

First, under Bondurant's leadership, the medical center was consolidated into four sectors:* the biomedical graduate research organization (BGRO), which coordinates the basic science departments and research in the clinical departments; the Lombardi Comprehensive Cancer Center; the school of medicine; and the school of nursing and health studies.

The BGRO, the arrival of which many of the basic scientists did not receive with enthusiasm,[16] coordinates all research and graduate medical education in the school of medicine, with the single exception of the Lombardi Comprehensive Cancer Center, the director of which, like that of the BGRO, reports directly to the executive vice president.[17] Georgetown created the BGRO for several purposes: to manage research more effectively within the school, improve training for those taking the graduate degrees of master and Ph.D., and reduce expenses by consolidating overlapping administrative functions.[14,18]

In the new organization, the chairmen of the five basic science departments† report administratively to Vassilios Papadopoulos,‡ the director of the BGRO, as does the associate dean for graduate education, who works closely with the dean of the graduate school of arts and sciences at the university. About 40 percent of the clinical faculty, whether employed by MedStar or the university, relate to the BGRO for the research they perform, with the clinical chairs reporting to the BGRO director for issues related to the research enterprise in their departments.[18]

The authority given to the director of the BGRO has, in effect, converted it from a staff job, called associate dean for research in many medical schools, into a position with line authority. The change introduced a level

---

*Also called "towers" and "silos," both names the administration does not favor.[7] "Let me explain why I use the sector concept rather than silo," says Dr. Ray Mitchell, the dean for medical education. "I believe the divisions are porous enough to create a true matrix organization. For example, I must purchase my educational product across all four sectors, [including] undergraduate medical and overlapping graduate programs."[15]

†Biochemistry and molecular and cellular biology; microbiology and immunology; neuroscience; pharmacology; and physiology and biophysics.[18]

‡Papadopoulos, former chairman of the department of biochemistry and molecular biology, left Georgetown in 2007 to become director of the research institute at McGill University Health Centre. He was succeeded as interim director of the BGRO by Dr. Robert Clarke from the Lombardi Cancer Center.

of administration, not present in most medical schools, between the basic science chairs and the executive dean. "This, in effect, minimized the fiscal responsibility of the chairs, thus reducing their academic powers," comments basic scientist Martin Morad.[19]

The chairmen of the departments of biostatistics, bioinformatics, and biomathematics; oncology; pathology; and radiation medicine report to Dr. Anatoly Dritschilo, the interim director of the Lombardi Comprehensive Cancer Center, for education and research and to MedStar for clinical affairs. Dritschilo, Mitchell, Papadopoulos, and Bette Keltner, the dean of the school of nursing and health studies, report to Bondurant. All department chairmen report for senior university affairs to Bondurant.

Despite the loss of the hospital and practice plan, Georgetown continues to refer to its medical enterprise as a "medical center," though the constituent parts are not organized as they are in most academic medical centers. There is the medical school, administratively referred to as "the office of the dean for medical education," whose primary responsibility is the selection of and education of the students. Research and the training of investigators are assigned to the BGRO. Lombardi is a separate entity as is, of course, the school of nursing and health studies.

The medical center treats the finances of each of these four units separately. With this method of accounting, only the research enterprise loses money. The salaries and benefits of the research faculty are its largest costs, and income from grants and endowments is insufficient to pay for them.

As for the budget, the losses of 2006 are on schedule to be reduced during 2007.[14] "Dramatic" amounts of money, however, have not yet been saved, according to Papadopoulos, "but BGRO's been around for less than a year," he said in the spring of 2006. "We have had some savings on expenses."[18] Spiros Dimolitsas, the chief administrative officer at the university who participated in restructuring the medical center, believes that revenue to solve the financial problems will come from better fundraising, increased revenue from licensing, and, eventually, contributions from the clinical enterprise.[20]

Committee Governance

In addition to the medical center caucus of the university faculty senate, both of which are seen as quite influential at Georgetown,[14] there are two major governance committees within the medical center.[21] The Executive Committee of twenty-three voting members and seven nonvoting members consists of, among others, selected and elected chairmen and faculty members of departments and centers, appointees from the faculty senate, a representative of the main campus, and, from MedStar, Joy Drass, the hospital CEO, and William Thomas, executive vice president for medical affairs.[22] The meeting is chaired by Bondurant or his designee. This is the group that approves promotions and nominations to executive positions,[23] but is otherwise seen as "not a deliberative body. It meets for an hour or an hour-and-a-half a month, with most of the time devoted to reports."[22]

In the Council of Chairs, the membership consists of each of the twenty-five department chairmen, two deans, and one director.[24] This group elects its chairman for a two-year term, with the position rotating between a clinical chairman and a basic-science chairman. Sam Wiesel is the current (2006) chairman.* This committee is, in Wiesel's words, "just advisory to the dean [who is an invited guest] with no real responsibility."[25] Another clinical chairman compares these sessions with those before MedStar, "when we actually made decisions."[26]

Faculty Tracks

Two years after MedStar bought the hospital and practice plan, the university revised the titles of faculty in the clinical departments who had become MedStar employees. They were originally designed for former university clinical faculty who practiced at Georgetown University Hospital. Now these tracks are used for clinicians who practice at any Georgetown affiliate and who may not be employed by the university. Georgetown also developed a new track for full-time university-employed faculty.[27-29]

The list below includes the different tracks as of January 2007, with the number of faculty in each track given parenthetically. At the time, Georgetown employed 223 members of the clinical faculty; 1,273 were employed by MedStar and other organizations or were practicing privately.

---

*Wiesel seems to have recovered from the low esteem in which he was held by the basic scientists previously. He is now, according to dean Mitchell, "very well respected, particularly among clinical chairs, [and] increasingly among basic chairs as the nature and significance of the financial challenges become clearer in retrospect, [and] the success of the hospital and the merger itself have become clearer."[15]

MedStar employees, none of whom are eligible for Georgetown tenure:

- *Clinician scholar* track (162) recognizes "faculty who make substantial and sustained contributions to the educational and research missions of Georgetown University School of Medicine in addition to providing service to the medical center and medical community." Their titles read, for example, "professor of medicine."
- *Clinical educator* track (199) recognizes "faculty who make important and continuing contributions to the education of Georgetown students, residents, and fellows and to others in the medical field, in addition to providing exemplary clinical care and service." Their titles read, for example, "professor of clinical medicine."
- *Clinician* track (870) recognizes "faculty who make sustained, but limited contributions to the education of trainees at the Georgetown University Medical Center, in addition to providing clinical care and service to the medical community. This track is intended primarily for individuals who are in private practice and who formerly would have been called 'voluntary' or 'part-time' faculty." Their titles read, for example, "clinical professor of medicine."

University employees:

- *Tenure* track (88 with tenure, 54 tenure track) recognizes "Georgetown University faculty who make substantial and sustained contributions to the scholarly mission in the areas of research, education, service and, if appropriate, patient care. It is intended for those who remain dedicated to the creation and dissemination of knowledge based upon original research related to basic investigations of normal biologic processes or diseases, clinical research, or medical education." Their titles read, for example, "professor of medicine" or "professor of microbiology and immunology."
- *Medical educator* track (15), a new non-tenure track, is "intended for university-employed medical school faculty members whose primary academic contributions are to teaching or other areas related to medical education and who held faculty appointments on tracks that have now been eliminated. . . . New appointments on the medical educator track will be for a limited number of faculty whose pri-

mary contributions are to teaching or other areas related to medical education." Their official titles read, for example, "assistant professor of medicine on the medical educator track." For external purposes, including grant applications and other university publications, the qualifier "on the medical educator track" may be dropped.

- *Research* track (148) is designed for full-time, non-tenure track faculty whose primary responsibilities are to "research programs [and may have] responsibilities toward training." Their "salaries are derived from specifically designated funds, including research grants and external funds." Their titles read, for example, "assistant professor of microbiology and immunology on the research track."

Research

Research at Georgetown medicine had long languished in both basic and clinical science.[14]* However, says Alan Faden, "given the small size of the basic science faculty and the smaller percentage of clinical research dollars as compared to peer institutions, productivity of the faculty has been relatively high."[31]

In 2005, the National Institutes of Health (NIH) ranked Georgetown sixtieth of 123 schools in the amount of awards.[32] In the medical center, only Stuart Bondurant, the interim executive vice president, and two members of the emeritus faculty are members of the Institute of Medicine.[33]† No one in the Georgetown medical faculty is a member of the National Academy of Sciences.[33] Because the medical center accounts for about 80 percent of all the research support in the university, "the university leadership loves this side of us," said one of the senior faculty.[34]

Current and former faculty members give several opinions to explain the medical school's modest research enterprise:[7,26,35-41]

*Bondurant comments: "This is compared with other institutions which are more strongly research based—we have never been primarily research focused so this is a somewhat unfair characterization. GUMC [Georgetown University Medical Center]–sponsored research dollars have consistently gone up from $77.3 million in fiscal year 1993 (earliest year I could get numbers) to $133.5 million in fiscal year 2006."[30]

† Two of the institute members in the medical school were elected before coming to Georgetown while they were working at other schools. Three members of the Georgetown University faculty in schools other than medicine are also members of the Institute of Medicine.[33]

- "Georgetown medicine has always been on a shoestring for research, no state money and tuition's the main source of revenue."
- "Since Griffith, none of the [permanent] executive vice presidents has had an academic vision or has emphasized academic excellence as a centerpiece."
- "Lack of research dollars means less money from indirects."

Many faculty believe that the merger with MedStar has injured rather than facilitated research at Georgetown.

- "MedStar doesn't fundamentally favor research."
- "The MedStar lawyers are concerned about what patients in research could mean. They're afraid of their own shadows."
- "Research has suffered because clinical faculty have less time for it."
- "It's almost killed it in my department. If you try to do research, you earn less money."
- "There's no focus in the culture on research and teaching. The e-mails from MedStar have to do only with clinical issues."

Alan Faden* explains. "Strategic changes at Georgetown University Medical Center have often been difficult to achieve. The environment provides few meaningful incentives for the successful investigator or teacher. There are very few endowed chairs, and there have been inadequate resources to recruit members of the National Academy of Sciences or Institute of Medicine. Finally, recruitment has often been piecemeal, without a strategic underlying vision to develop regional centers of excellence that could enhance recruitment of both faculty and patients."[42]

"The climate for clinical research has not improved much," Stuart Bondurant admits.[14] Other members of the faculty agree,[7,26,43-46] while some believe it has worsened.[38,47-50] Basic scientists complain that preoccupation with fulfilling the clinical goals set by MedStar prevents members of the clinical faculty from collaborating with the basic scientists as much as before the merger.[49] So long as the dual lines of authority govern the relationship, Georgetown's standing among the nation's research-intensive medical schools will continue to lag, one former chairman predicted.[47]

---

*Faden (B.A., Pennsylvania; M.D., Chicago) trained in neurology at the University of California, San Francisco (UCSF), and held faculty positions at the Uniformed Services University of the Health Sciences in Bethesda, Maryland, and at UCSF (vice chairman, department of neurology) before coming to Georgetown in 1991 as dean of research and graduate education and scientific director of the medical center.

Basic Science

To help improve research productivity in the midst of significant financial limitations, the university has reorganized the basic science departments, first by combining the department of cell biology with biochemistry and molecular biology.* Budgets would now be based on scientific programs rather than on departments. Although not the only measure considered,[52] success in obtaining grants would determine, more often than in the past, the compensation of the scientific faculty.[18,53] "The basic scientists didn't understand how precarious the medical school had become," said Paul Katz, chairman of the department of medicine from 1997 to 2001. "They continuously fought the school's basing lab space on productivity."[37] For the moment, further reorganization has been postponed.[18]

The chairmen have lost the authority to assign space or hire faculty because most of their former administrative duties have been assumed by the BGRO. "Dr. Bondurant called us [basic science chairmen] into his office one Friday," remembers Martin Dym, then the chairman of cell biology, "and told us that all our administrators would be fired on Monday.† We were furious."[53] Although more than half of the discharged workers were immediately rehired, they would now report to the dean for medical education or the director of the BGRO, no longer to the chairs.[53] As a result of these changes, the school reduced its losses and centralized its administrative structure, but not without pain.

With "the basic sciences departments now departments in name only," according to Michael Lumpkin, former chairman of the department of physiology and biophysics,[34] some of the basic science chairmen resigned during 2005, in some cases not discouraged from doing so by Bondurant.[18] They have been replaced by chairmen on three-year contracts,[18] who were willing to take on what Lumpkin sees as "administrative responsibili-

---

*In 2004, the NIH ranked the Georgetown basic science departments (number of schools with such departments and percentile among those schools in parentheses):[51] biochemistry and molecular and cellular biology—83 (109, 76 percent), microbiology and immunology—62 (103, 60 percent), neuroscience—19 (32, 59 percent), pharmacology—40 (101, 40 percent), physiology and biophysics—77 (98, 79 percent).

†"If 'fired' means discharged, it is incorrect since all the employees he is referring to were given two months' notice and offered other positions (which all but two accepted) and are still employed in them," Bondurant explains.[54]

ties with minimal authority to act."[34]* Each was appointed from current Georgetown faculty without national searches.[18]

"Although the role of the chairs is different," Papadopoulos says, "it remains vital and central to the function of BGRO and the institution."[55] Bondurant sees the changes as "a carefully planned, well-orchestrated, and successful transition."[30]

The freeze on recruiting leaves only two of the twelve faculty members untenured in physiology and biophysics.† When they achieve tenure or leave, the department will have no younger members in the tenure track. "We're headed into mediocrity from which it will be very difficult to escape," warns Lumpkin. "Cohesiveness and camaraderie are falling as we realize that building new programs is becoming nearly impossible."[34] With the number of productive faculty in the basic sciences decreasing and laboratories becoming vacant, the school of medicine has leased a floor in one of its buildings to the chemistry department in the college.

Members of the basic science departments express their displeasure with much of what has happened:

- "There's malaise among us."
- "We're starting to feel like factory workers."
- "The structure couldn't be more destructive."
- "It was a way to castrate the chairs."
- "They took away all the money we had saved in our discretionary accounts."

A former member of the department of physiology with a somewhat different view of its problems is Martin Morad, whom John Griffith recruited to Georgetown as chairman from the University of Pennsylvania in 1994. On arriving, Morad found the department poorly funded from the NIH. He tried to motivate the faculty to get involved in new projects that would have higher likelihood of success and fundability. "I want you all on a fast train with many new and exciting young scientists," he told his new colleagues. To Griffith, he said, "This is a boutique place. You should combine the departments into institutes."

Morad resigned from the chair and considered returning to Penn after the

---

*When I visited Lumpkin, he was in the process of moving out of what had been the chairman's office to a smaller space near his laboratory. He pointed to the unoccupied desks of the department's former secretary and administrator, positions that had been eliminated.[34]

†In the winter of 2006.

impasse between him and the faculty became insurmountable—"I wasn't politically savvy," he acknowledges[56]—but his wife, a lawyer, preferred living in Washington. Griffith supported Morad's decision to stay and transferred his appointment to the more research-oriented and better-endowed department of pharmacology, where he continues his well-funded research. "The faculty in physiology wanted a teaching and not a research department. They have prospered doing just that!" Morad says.[56]*

Although the university does not require that faculty doing research assign a fraction of their grants to their salaries, as many research-intensive medical schools do, "the medical center strongly encourages all faculty who are involved in research to maintain at least 50 percent of their salary on research and research track faculty are expected to have more than 75 percent of their salaries on research," Bondurant explains.[30]

This has led to conflict between research faculty in the clinical departments, who believe that they have a greater responsibility to develop salary support than some of the basic science investigators. "There was a feeling by the clinical faculty that the basic scientists were not putting forth a good faith effort to respond to the financial challenges of the school," said Daniel Clauw, former chief of the rheumatology division and vice chairman of the department of medicine. "They believed in a socialist system—got their salaries, their historical allotments of space, etc.—whereas the clinical faculty were quite accustomed to being held accountable for their salaries and paying for their overhead because this was expected in the clinical care enterprise. In fact, the clinical faculty in general were supportive of moving to a more entrepreneurial system."[57] While clinicians like Clauw held the basic scientists responsible for the losses, the basic scientists blamed the hospital and the practice plan.[58] One of the problems, explained one of the former basic science chairmen, was "we were never challenged from the top."[53]

The chairman who did not resign is Kenneth Dretchen, who, like several chairmen in this time of financial troubles, had been appointed to the pharmacology chair without a national search.† What pharmacology has

---

*Martin Morad is a highly accomplished scientist in cardiovascular biology, with over 200 peer reviewed publications, 20 of which are published in *Science* magazine. In his career he has trained over 80 colleagues, 11 of whom have become chiefs or chairmen of departments in U.S., European, and Japanese medical schools.[56]

† As of the summer of 2006, only two chairmen in the clinical departments had been chosen through a national search. When the Liaison Committee on Medical Education (LCME) was preparing to visit Georgetown, the school decided that having so many interim chairmen—as many as seven at one point—would not create the most attractive impression. Consequently, most of them

that the other basic science departments, or what is left of them, do not have is its own money. The university established an endowment for the department that included the proceeds from a fund, now worth $8 million, that was developed from the patent rights to a drug invented in the department when Dr. Raymond Woosley was chairman.* In addition, Dretchen holds a $2 million endowed chair created by a pharmaceutical house several decades ago. Accordingly, he has been recently able to recruit five tenure-track investigators.[35]

Dretchen continues to control his space and budget, although, administratively, pharmacology and microbiology share some functions. Despite keeping most of his own independence, he acknowledges that "it's harder to maintain cohesiveness, particularly in the weaker departments."[35]

The merger with MedStar has caused Dretchen and some of his colleagues[49] at least one problem, recruiting junior members of the clinical departments to teach the students in his pharmacology course. "They're under such pressure to practice." Some senior faculty who teach in Dretchen's courses, however, continue to do so. They believe that "if you wear the Georgetown emblem, there's no job you won't do. So what happens when the senior people leave?"[35]

This problem, however, is not universal among the basic sciences. The surgeons and radiologists who teach anatomy continue to do so despite their conversion into MedStar employees. Perhaps the reason for this is that the surgeons and radiologists consider anatomy central to their discipline.[53] In their monthly meetings the chairmen discuss, among other topics, how to collaborate in such matters.[53]

The Medical Center versus the University

In 2001, Georgetown University elected John J. DeGioia its forty-eighth president, the first layman to lead the university. DeGioia is Georgetown personified. He received his B.A. in English and Ph.D. in philosophy there and has worked and taught at Georgetown throughout his career.† Like

---

were converted to permanent status, some with limited three-year contracts, and each with the assent of the members of the relevant departments.[59]

*Woosley subsequently became dean of the school of medicine at the University of Arizona and is now president and chief executive officer of the Critical Path Institute, Tucson, Arizona.

†His wife is also a Georgetown graduate.

Stephen Trachtenberg at George Washington, DeGioia is primarily an academic administrator. Described as "very astute politically, meticulous, and careful," DeGioia is seen as "conflict-averse." Before becoming president, DeGioia was the university's senior vice president and intimately involved in the sale of the hospital and practice plan.

"A large part of the difficulties historically arose because of a unique dysfunctional relationship between the medical center and the university," believes Kenneth Bloem, former CEO of the medical center. "There was confusion at the ultimate levels of governance, by senior Georgetown directors, those serving on committees like finance and the committee for the medical center."[60] He is not alone in this opinion. Many now or formerly in the medical school hold the directors on Georgetown University's board of directors and particularly the members of the health affairs committee responsible for the medical center's decade of troubles.[22,61-63] Some believe that the board's inadequate supervision of the medical center was the basic problem. "It's an honorific, not a governing group," several observers have said in so many words.

Bloem holds that the central university administration, not so much the directors, exercised too much control—"interference" he would call it—rather than too little. "The university should have disengaged itself from dominating the hospital so it could be responsible for its own problems. This wasn't possible because the university staff didn't want to give up control."[60]

Gary Filerman, chairman of the department of health systems administration in the school of nursing and health studies, says, "The boards lack expertise in the realities of academic health in general and academic health centers in particular. They are subject to mythologies, such as the notion that all such centers lose money, and may not even apply what they do know about effective management such as the need to align responsibility with authority. In our case, it appears that the full dimensions of the financial and organizational problems were not appreciated for years."[22] Filerman thinks part of the problem is due to the fact that "many boards don't have agendas and information beyond what the university officers give them, and all too often, do not ask the hard questions."[22] In particular, according to one of the medical center's financial executives, the directors did not understand how much the hospital was subsidizing the university.[36]

Jesuit Influence

The Jesuit leadership of Georgetown University has affected the development of medicine at Georgetown negatively in the opinion of several members of the medical faculty. When the dental school closed, President Healy,
it was rumored, discussed with his advisors closing the medical school
also.* They rejected this proposal for financial and programmatic reasons.
The expenses during the closing would have been unsupportable: paying
the tenure of the faculty, resolving debts on the buildings, operating the
school as the tuitions decreased. Furthermore, closing the school was not
the appropriate decision for Georgetown, which prided itself on being a
comprehensive, national research university with a Jesuit mission of service
as well as education.[64]

A particularly knowledgeable observer of Georgetown medicine's trials
and successes is Dr. Edwin ("Ned") Cassem, a psychiatrist and Jesuit priest
who works at the Massachusetts General Hospital in Boston. Cassem was
chairman of his department there for twelve years, is a professor in the
Harvard Medical School, and was a member of the Georgetown University
board of directors, except for one year, from 1990 to 2004.†

Cassem senses "an incredible ambivalence" among Jesuit leaders about
building strong medical schools. Though very well educated in other fields,
few Jesuits become physicians—Cassem is a notable exception—or have
acquired advanced degrees in the medical sciences.[65]

Many in the medical school believe that the Jesuits who have led Georgetown were more committed to undergraduate than to graduate or professional education and more oriented to humanistic studies, like history,
religion, and languages, than to medical science.[66]‡ Laboratories cost
money, and in Georgetown's case, with its small endowment, less expensive
academic programs often take precedence.[66] What fundraising the university conducted emphasized the college and law school. The medical school
has never had an effective development office of its own,[64] and the univer-

---

*University officials deny that Father Healy considered closing the medical school.[8]

†Cassem's M.D. is from Harvard, not Georgetown.

‡Dr. Bondurant adds, "They built at Georgetown one of the top five law schools in the country
and arguably the best school of foreign service in the world, both far beyond basic undergraduate
education."[54]

sity did little to encourage such activity despite the presence of patients grateful to the faculty for their care, a source of philanthropy employed with much success at other academic medical centers.[67]*

The Jesuits' dedication to, as Cassem puts it, "the good and well-being of the whole person—body, mind, and spirit"[69]—means that "service usually trumps academics"[70] when a Catholic institution has to decide whether to recruit an expensive scientific or medical investigator or fund a free clinic. "Giving a high priority to medical research would decrease our emphasis on mission," Cassem said. "However, we never acted this way about pure science. Most Jesuits respect the Ph.D. more than the M.D."[69]

The data from fiscal year 2005 support these statements.[32] Each of the four U.S. Jesuit medical schools rank relatively low in research support from the NIH when compared with 123 U.S. medical schools: Creighton 116, Loyola-Stritch 89, and St. Louis 80. Georgetown has the most NIH support among the Jesuit schools but still ranks only 60th.†

Future Leadership

Since Sam Wiesel returned to full-time orthopedics from the positions of executive vice president and executive dean in 2002, the school has been led for two terms by an interim leader, Stuart Bondurant, and by Dr. Daniel Sedmak, a pathologist from Ohio State University who held the position on a permanent, albeit short-lived, basis from July 2003 to August 2004. Sedmak had begun to reduce the losses, but, according to several observers, insufficiently to satisfy his employers, so he left Georgetown and returned to Columbus.‡

In the spring of 2006, the university formed a search committee to find a permanent vice president/executive dean. No searches for permanent department chairmen are being conducted until this appointment is made.

Now that MedStar runs the Georgetown University Hospital and the

---

*Some worry about competition between MedStar, which controls the clinical enterprise, and the medical school for contributions from grateful patients.[43,68]

†From 1970 to 2005, the NIH ranked Georgetown from a high of 40 (1977, 34th percentile) to a low of 71 (1981, 56th percentile).[71] During the recent years of trouble, its rank has fallen from 45 in 1999, the year before the sale to MedStar, to 63 in 2004; there was improvement in 2005 (it rose to 60th).[10,32] The amount of support for research from other agencies and from industry has risen recently.[10]

‡Dr. Sedmak declined to be interviewed for this book.

faculty's practice group, the role and, consequently, the prominence of the executive vice president, like his counterpart at George Washington, has shrunk.[12] His direct responsibilities are limited to education and research in the medical school and overseeing the school of nursing and health studies. Consequently, some have suggested that Georgetown could appoint a basic scientist to the position. If this happens, should the title of executive vice president be retired and the senior officer in the medical school be called dean again? Under such a reorganization, the dean of the school of nursing and health studies might then report directly to the president.

Bondurant, who sees Georgetown as "a very conservative, faculty-driven place,"[14] thinks this approach unwise. He and others[7] believe that his successor will have more responsibilities than only supervising education and research in the medical school. The interim executive vice president sees the incumbent active "within the university . . . and with outside entities such as hospital systems and federal agencies, not for prestige but operationally to represent the complex. There is a real building job to be done beyond the operation of the schools. The relation to MedStar offers great potential promise to Georgetown if knowledgably managed and great potential problems if not well managed."[72]

Alan Faden, the senior, well-funded investigative neurologist who was dean of research and graduate education and scientific director of the medical center in John Griffith's administration, agrees. "Georgetown needs an executive vice president who will recognize both our research and clinical needs and be capable of building bridges and collaborations."[31]

Bondurant hopes that in the near future* he will be able to return to the retirement from which Georgetown twice called him. But there are special problems in the recruitment of his successor. How will candidates react to the history of frequent changes in the office during the past decade? Does this reflect conflict, which may be continuing, between the medical center and the university administration? How many top-flight candidates will take a job at a medical school with few resources, currently in a precarious financial condition, and how many academic clinicians would be interested when the medical school does not own at least some part of the clinical enterprise?

Some think that a current faculty member may be the only person that

---

*Comments made in 2006.

Georgetown can appoint at this time. Bondurant, however, believes that a highly competent candidate from outside can be found but agrees that academics from clinical departments may have reservations. "It's in Med-Star's interest to have a person they can work with. I believe our working relations are even now a partnership in several material ways. There are substantial resources there."[72]

"We will leverage location, tradition, values, and our global network to assure that we recruit an excellent executive vice president and that the medical center thrives," said Georgetown president Jack DeGioia.[73]

Stuart Bondurant's Successor

Georgetown overcame the reservations of skeptics on its faculty by announcing on November 29, 2006, the appointment of Howard J. Federoff, M.D., Ph.D., as executive vice president for health sciences and executive dean of the school of medicine, effective April 1, 2007.[74] When recruited from the University of Rochester School of Medicine, Federoff was senior associate dean for basic research; professor of genetics, immunology, medicine, microbiology, neurology, and oncology; and founding director of the center for aging and development biology at the institute of biomedical sciences at Rochester.

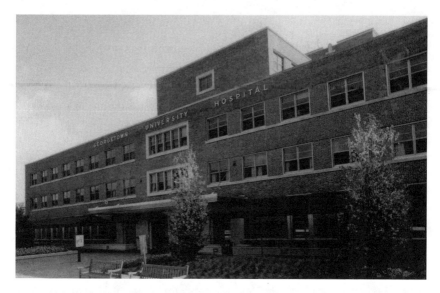

The Georgetown University Hospital, which MedStar Health bought in 2000. *Courtesy of MedStar Health.*

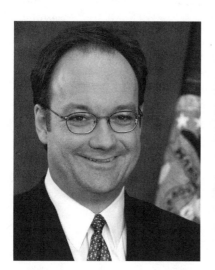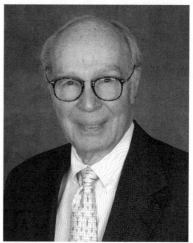

John ("Jack") DeGioia (*left*), president of Georgetown University and its first leader who is not a Jesuit priest. Dr. Stuart Bondurant (*right*), the experienced academic physician who was twice drafted from retirement as interim executive vice president of the medical center. *Courtesy of Georgetown University.*

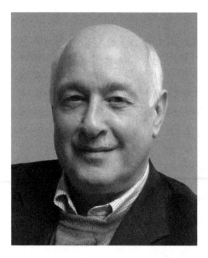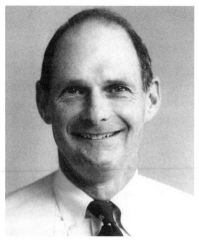

Kenneth Bloem (*left*), CEO of the medical center from 1996 to 1999, whom the university hired to try to repair its financial and operational problems. Dr. Sam Wiesel (*right*), the orthopedist who helped engineer the transition after MedStar purchased the hospital and practice plan, an effort that brought him heartache from some of his colleagues on the faculty. *Photo of Kenneth Bloem courtesy of Kenneth Bloem; photo of Sam Wiesel courtesy of Georgetown University*

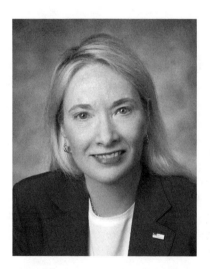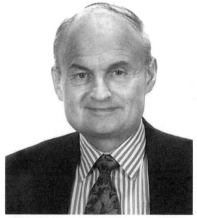

Dr. Joy Drass (*left*), the internist-CEO and Georgetown medical school alumna who led the financial turnaround of the Georgetown University Hospital. Previously, Drass was an executive at the Washington Hospital Center. Dr. Edwin ("Ned") Cassem (*right*), the Jesuit psychiatrist from Harvard who was a Georgetown trustee when MedStar bought the hospital and practice plan. *Photo of Joy Drass courtesy of MedStar Health; photo of Edwin Cassem courtesy of Edwin Cassem*

CHAPTER NINE

MedStar Health

MedStar Health is the name of a not-for-profit hospital system that in 2000 acquired the Georgetown University Hospital. Its origins reach back into the history of several community hospitals in Baltimore and Washington.

Franklin Square Hospital Tries to Meet the Challenges of Managed Care

The coming of managed care challenged the leaders of America's hospitals, great and small. Franklin Square Hospital, a medium-sized community hospital in Baltimore, tried several schemes in its attempts to compete successfully.

Founded by eight physicians in 1898 as the National Temperance Hospital of Baltimore City, the hospital soon moved and adopted the name of the park in West Baltimore that it faced. Like several hospitals in Baltimore and many cities, Franklin Square found itself by the 1960s in a depressed, deteriorating part of the city. Faced with the challenge of modernizing an aging facility as well as competing with two other recently established hospitals in the same area, the trustees decided to move Franklin Square to east Baltimore County, into a rapidly growing community with no hospital. A new plant was constructed, and although the new hospital in a new location opened in 1969, the original name was retained despite the hospital's having moved far from its earlier location. By 2005, Franklin Square Hospital had 329 beds, 850 physicians on its staff, and several residency training programs.

In the mid-1980s, in advance of many hospitals, Franklin Square and several members of its medical staff created their own preferred provider organization (PPO) and health maintenance organization (HMO) and, in association with five other local community hospitals,[1] consolidated these ventures into the Preferred Health Network (PHN) to try to weather the new world of managed care. As Franklin Square CEO Michael Merson* described the venture, "We were organizing to deliver low-cost best practice care with doctors who wanted to be involved in managed care."[1]

Soon, the hospital's board and Merson, recognizing that running an insurance venture was an activity for which they were inadequately experienced, sold a controlling interest in these ventures to an out-of-state company. By 1999, Blue Cross/Blue Shield of Maryland had bought PHN, including all the hospitals' holdings. PHN had lost money each year before the Blues took over.[1]

These efforts convinced the Franklin Square leaders that creating a regional network of hospitals would give them the best opportunity of negotiating successfully with the insurers for patients by becoming indispensable to payers, "whoever they may be," Merson said.[1] They assumed that large employers would prefer working with a regional network, which would offer patients greater choice of where they would receive their medical care, than with individual hospitals.

Securing higher rates from the carriers was less easily accomplished in Maryland than in other states because of the state's Health Services Cost Review Commission (HSCRC), which established the rates hospitals would receive from all payers.[3] The HSCRC provides a safety net for well-run hospitals in Maryland by assuring that they can make at least some surplus— much less than the hospitals want, of course—"but discourages one trying to be the best," according to Merson. "We saw ourselves severely con-

---

*Called by one of his admirers "a visionary, several years ahead of most people."[2]

strained by the rate regulation system. We wanted to create our own vision of our future in spite of regulated rates."[1] With the hospital's leaders unable to affect rates, they concentrated on how to make sure that the patients subscribing to particular insurance products would come to Franklin Square. All this planning was predicated on how the executives and board thought managed care would evolve.[1]

Helix

Before creating a successful merger, Franklin Square had negotiated unsuccessfully with two hospitals. In one case, the board decided not to continue, and in the other, the CEO of the hospital scuttled the deal at the last minute when it became clear that Merson would become CEO of the merged company.[1]

Union Memorial Hospital then became available. Located at the junction of one of the more depressed areas of downtown Baltimore to the south and the high-income suburbs to the north and close to the arts and sciences campus of Johns Hopkins University, Union had a long and valued history of providing medical care to Baltimoreans.* The seven women who founded it 150 years ago to provide care for "the sick, the poor, and the infirm" named it the Union Protestant Infirmary.

By 2005, Union would have 283 licensed beds and 656 physicians on its staff, and, although it was not in the best financial shape in the mid-1980s, Union had made a bid to buy a small community hospital that was converting from for-profit to not-for-profit status. Although the attempt failed, the leaders of Union had revealed that the hospital was available for a merger of some sort. "Union was not our first choice," says Merson. "We would have preferred to go with one of the hospitals in our PHN [Preferred Health Network], and Union was not a member."[1]

Merson observes that deciding with which hospital to merge is "pretty speculative. You can't predict. It's so idiosyncratic."[1] In this case, joining Franklin Square with Union would constitute a merger "with no money," as Dr. William Thomas, then chairman of the department of medicine at Franklin Square, said. "We were making a bit, Union was in the red."[2] Nev-

---

* "Baltimorons" to some.

ertheless, if the hospitals could come together, it would constitute Baltimore's "first real merger."[2]

As the negotiations proceeded, at least one problem that had killed an earlier merger attempt was not applicable with Union. The CEO was about to retire, and he and Merson agreed that the Union chief would be CEO of the merged corporation for a year, and then Merson would take over. A New York firm helped the leaders find a suitable name for the new company, and after many attempts, decided on Helix. "No one else was using it, and most people knew of its relation to medical science," explains Merson.[1]

Merging the two hospitals in 1987 was relatively easy compared with what followed during the first years of Helix's existence. The structure of the new board was a leading problem. The membership consisted of three trustees each from the boards of Franklin Square and Union hospitals with Merson, now the CEO of Helix, the member "to break any ties," as he puts it.[1] Thus, each of the board members had been affiliated with one of the hospitals; there were no outside members. "It was tough for some of the board members to take off their original hats," explains Merson. Though he had resigned as CEO of Franklin Square when he became CEO of Helix, Merson was seen as partial to his old hospital, in part, because he had brought several of his associates from Franklin Square to fill the executive offices at Helix. "This went on for four years, during what I would call the first generation of Helix."[1]*

Franklin Square, which had made a surplus of $4.6 million for the year ending June 30, 1993, had merged with a hospital that had lost $950,000 during the same period, which was Union's fourth year of operating losses.[5] "The culture at Union," according to Merson, "was far more problematic. We knew that Union was troubled financially." Franklin Square, however, did not have the cash to rescue Union, so "we needed to fix them," a process that took four years until Union generated a surplus.

This was not a happy time. "There were a lot of social problems," Thomas said, proving that "medicine is tribal."[2] Union CEOs came and went, and

*This problem, equal number of board members from the founding institutions on the board of the merged company, was one of the reasons that the merger of the hospitals of the University of California, San Francisco, and Stanford University failed after only twenty-three months. The three outside board members were outnumbered by twelve inside trustees—six from each hospital and medical school. The groups from each institution caucused in advance of board meetings to decide how they would approach issues in the best interest of their institutions.[4]

the staff and doctors became frustrated. Much of the animus was directed toward Merson, the CEO from a competing hospital. "The problem over me led to a crisis on the board," Merson remembers.[1]

At this point, Merson was approached by two relatively weak hospitals interested in joining Helix. Merson, however, was more interested in another, and asked the smaller hospitals to "back off"[1] for the time being. The hospital Merson favored was Good Samaritan.[5,6]

Good Samaritan Hospital Joins Helix

"Good Sam" had been one of Merson's first choices when Helix was being created, but its board and executives were not interested then. By 1994, when Good Samaritan became Helix's third hospital, market forces were changing and Good Sam was being inundated by low-income patients as the character of its community changed. The hospital's leadership also thought that being part of a larger group would attract business from managed care companies, which, as Michael Merson said, "want to deal with one entity. We made a value judgment that the future was in systems. As a single hospital we would not be able to negotiate with third-party payers—the HMOs. We wouldn't be able to provide a full range of services."[1]

Despite the potential problems its leaders envisioned, Good Samaritan had many attractive features. It had 287 licensed beds, a 137-bed nursing home, a 94-unit elderly housing complex, 2 medical office buildings[6] and what Merson saw as a good administration and a highly ethical board. Merson knew and admired the chief operating officer and chief financial officer. Financially, Merson believed Good Sam to be "the best-managed hospital in the state." It had no debt and $100 million in cash and investments.[1]* The addition of Good Samaritan would bring to Helix a total of 1,080 licensed hospital beds and 239 nursing home beds.[5] No cash changed hands in the merger into Helix of both Union and Good Samaritan hospitals. Helix assumed the debt of both institutions as it had for Franklin Square.

The incorporation of Good Samaritan did, however, introduce an important administrative change. James ("Jim") Oakey, the Good Sam CEO, replaced Michael Merson as head of Helix. The conflict between Merson and

*Johns Hopkins Hospital was also interested in acquiring Good Samaritan. The conflict between the dean of the medical school and the hospital president at the time[7] extended to this potential deal, and the much smaller and less prestigious Helix won the day.

the Union board members and doctors led to the Helix board's hiring a consultant who concluded that the cultural conflicts were too strong and advised that a leadership change would be wise.* The Helix board wanted to bring Good Samaritan into Helix with its absence of debt, charitable foundation, and other favorable features, but did not anticipate a favorable outcome in the midst of what Merson calls a "firefight" at Union. So Merson agreed to relinquish the position of CEO, and the Helix board concurred. Merson became vice chairman of the Helix board, a paid position but without much authority since the new CEO would report to the board chairman and not to him. The board insisted that Merson stay at Helix for at least three years.[8]

The addition of Good Samaritan dramatically strengthened Helix's financial situation by improving its balance sheet and increasing its ability to assume more debt. Trustees from Good Samaritan joined the Helix board, but the powers of the individual hospital boards decreased somewhat. Helix assumed all responsibility for strategy and finances, powers that had previously been also exercised by the hospital boards, leaving the hospital boards to emphasize quality of care and community issues.[8]

Church and Harbor Hospitals

Helix next combined with the Church Hospital, a long-established hospital and nursing home only two blocks from the Johns Hopkins medical campus. Church was losing a small amount of money each year, but had endowments and owned a large ambulatory center in the blue-collar community of Dundalk, a location important to Franklin Square because of its competition with the nearby Bayview Medical Center, the old city hospital

---

*Merson reads an important part of the conflict as reflecting the differences between the fundamental character of Union and Franklin Square. From its founding and until about fifteen years ago, the board of managers at Union consisted exclusively of women with a board of trustees of leading male citizens to advise the managers about financial and legal matters. Both groups reflected old-line Baltimore wealth and society. The same characteristics applied to many of its physicians, frequently graduates of the Johns Hopkins Hospital School of Medicine and/or its hospital's training programs. "I was from the other side of the tracks," Merson says as the former leader of a hospital located in an area of recent development and without the history and connections of Union and its leaders and doctors. Union doctors assumed that the physicians at Franklin Square would refer patients to them, one of the attractions to Union of the merger. This did not happen. Franklin Square had most of the services at Union, and most tellingly to Merson, the Union doctors would not visit Franklin Square and develop relationships with the doctors there.[8]

now owned by Johns Hopkins Health System.[8] A less obvious advantage for acquiring Church involved the state's desire to close some hospitals in this over-bedded region. Helix saw the possibility of eventually closing Church and receiving a bonus from the Health Services Cost Review Commission in increased rates at Union for the costs of performing this "public service." "Looking at all these things," observed Merson, "the Church deal didn't look so bad."[8] The cost to Helix to buy Church was $1 and absorption of its $30 million debt.*

The fifth and final hospital to be brought into Helix was the Harbor Hospital and its health system. Harbor was one of the hospitals that approached Michael Merson about a merger when Helix was negotiating with Good Samaritan in 1994. By November 1995, Helix was ready to incorporate Harbor, a 376-bed hospital in South Baltimore, into the Helix system.[9] Like so many other community hospital trustees and executives, Harbor's board had decided "that an independent hospital was unlikely to thrive in the long term," in the words of its chairman.[9] Without having merged with the healthy Good Samaritan, Helix would not have had the resources to obtain Church and Harbor hospitals.[8]

Helix Tries to Merge with the Johns Hopkins Hospital; Helix CEO Changes

On several occasions, the CEOs at Helix had tried to create some type of union with the Johns Hopkins Hospital. Merson had approached Hopkins hospital president James Block not long after Block arrived in Baltimore from Cleveland in 1992. "Jim and I knew each other from former contacts," Merson said. "We decided to keep it quiet until we saw if the boards were interested."[8] The Hopkins hospital board was not. Hopkins had been burned during a previous attempt to merge with two Baltimore community hospitals during the tenure of Robert Heyssel, Block's predecessor.[10] "Jim told me that the Hopkins culture would not allow doing another merger of that type. We're going to have to compete with you, but let's remain friends. End of discussion."[8]

---

*MedStar Health, Helix's successor, would eventually close Church and sell the buildings and property to the Johns Hopkins Hospital for $25 million. Hopkins traded the Church properties for a large tract of land owned by the Department of Housing and Urban Development (HUD) across the street from the Johns Hopkins Hospital and built a large parking garage there.

When Good Samaritan Hospital joined Helix, James Oakey, who had succeeded Michael Merson as CEO of Helix, approached the Hopkins hospital again. Good Samaritan had had a longstanding relationship with Hopkins. The medical school's orthopedics, rheumatology, and rehabilitation programs had been based there for decades. By 1997, when these talks took place, Block was gone and Dr. Edward Miller was the dean and CEO of the restructured Johns Hopkins Medicine, which included both the hospital and the medical school.[11] When Miller indicated an interest in discussing the possibilities, Oakey "brought the Helix board in," Merson remembers, and "described the union as a 'merger of equals,' "[8] an exaggeration, to say the least. The arrangement that Hopkins suggested was seen, particularly by the doctors at Union, as a Hopkins takeover, not the description of the merger Oakey had taken to his board.

Adding to Oakey's problems was the Helix balance sheet, which had deteriorated significantly because of the stock market's problems. Oakey had been buying physician practices at great expense and adopting risk in his managed care contracts. "We looked less financially secure," said Merson, who had advised against this strategy. Oakey had told Ed Miller that, to secure the merger, Helix, with its large cash reserves, would contribute $25 million per year to Hopkins, "the driver for me," as Miller describes his interest in the deal.[12] "A $25 million dollar a year donation to Hopkins to support education and research would be like receiving a $500 million gift. To have $25 million coming in year after year was not something to discard lightly."[13] The Johns Hopkins Medicine board saw the value of linking with a community hospital, particularly one with which it had a longstanding relationship, but was wary about the whole deal.[12]

"Jim [Oakey] had gotten caught up in his enthusiasm for the thing," Miller remembers. Oakey had not told the whole story to his board about important aspects of the deal with Hopkins, including the annual $25 million. "He thought he owned the board," Miller observed.[12] He did not, and, eventually, his board forced him to resign as Helix CEO.[8,12,14] "Oakey's credibility had vanished," according to Merson.[8]*

---

*Merson and Oakey brought different characteristics to the job of Helix CEO. Merson, more deliberative than Oakey,[15] was described, according to someone quoted in the *Baltimore Sun*, as "a methodical consensus builder, while Oakey was the opposite. . . . He wasn't the type to build consensus."[14] Oakey, described as blunt, earthy, flamboyant, even mercurial,[1] and a "character,"[16] once startled the staff at Good Samaritan, according to the *Sun*, "by loading his briefcase with 200 $1 bills

The Helix management caucused and advised the board to invite Merson to return as CEO. Back in his former job, Merson spoke with Miller at Hopkins because some of the Helix board favored trying one more time to link with Hopkins. Despite several meetings, which Merson describes as "excellent, we laid out what had gone right and wrong," the Johns Hopkins Medicine board maintained its position that such a merger was unwise for Hopkins, and consequently, the attempt to create a link between Helix and Hopkins failed for the third time.

Helix and Medlantic Merge; Medstar Created

Having failed so far to bring about a merger that Merson thought would be wise for Helix, he turned next to the Medlantic Healthcare Group in Washington. Merson first met the CEO of Medlantic, John McDaniel, when, as a junior administrator at Franklin Square, Merson was hospitalized at Maryland General Hospital, where McDaniel was a young administrator. In January 1982, McDaniel had become CEO of the Washington Hospital Center and later created the Medlantic Healthcare Group.

"I remember that John came to see me to ask how I was feeling and about my experience at his hospital," Merson said. "I saw this as an excellent way of conducting himself."[17] Merson and McDaniel became friends, and when Helix began to look at relationships outside the Baltimore area, Merson turned to Medlantic as a possible partner. "To become an indispensable provider, we needed to supply key services that no insurer could ignore and then leverage into the best contracts we could get." Merson believed that Helix had become too "urban centered" and owned no hospitals in suburban areas.[17]

Helix and Medlantic first formed a joint venture[18] that would have its own board consisting of executives from the two companies. By January 1996, the entity had been given a name, BWHealth, and had developed offices in Columbia, Maryland, midway between Baltimore and Washington.[19] An executive was recruited from a hospital system in California to be BWHealth's president and a small staff of twelve was appointed.[20] The alli-

---

and tossing them around the meeting room while telling the doctors, 'You know damn well I'm not interested in throwing money around.'"[14]

Michael Merson and Edward Miller supplied much of this narrative. I was unable to locate and interview James Oakey.

ance hoped to recruit patients from payers who worked in both the Baltimore and Washington markets. The leaders anticipated that BWHealth would:[18]

- Enable the constituent hospitals to avoid creating competitive services. Helix might send its cancer therapy patients to Medlantic's respected cancer facility. Medlantic would save the money to create its own hand trauma center because Helix already had one based at Union.
- Share the cost of building new primary care offices in surrounding counties of Maryland.
- Reduce patients' confusion when seeking different specialties of care since the new company would offer them all, although not necessarily at any one facility.
- Enable the estimated 150,000 people who commute between Baltimore and Washington to join a network offering care in both sites, even though parts of the alliance were as much as forty miles apart.
- Because of the size of the alliance, discourage other hospital-owning companies from trying to pick off any of the constituent parts.

Despite these attractive possibilities, BWHealth developed slowly and, as Merson saw it, was "spotty." James Oakey, the Helix CEO, had been concentrating on developing an eventually unsuccessful merger with the Hopkins hospital and was spending less time and energy on BWHealth. "There was a lot of angst because of a lack of progress," remembers Merson.[17]

By the fall of 1997, Oakey was gone, and Merson, back as Helix CEO, began talking with McDaniel about converting the "spotty" joint venture into a full asset merger. "He and I were very open with each other," Merson remembers. Oakey had bought many physician practices which, according to Merson, were "losing money big-time." Helix had sponsored a risk-contracting primary care network that was also losing money. Merson estimated that getting out of the practices and Helix's insurance vehicle could cost as much as $100 million or possibly more. Since Medlantic financial status was healthier—McDaniel, for example, had bought fewer practices—Helix had a strong financial incentive to merge with a less threatened entity like Medlantic.

Despite these financial problems, Helix would bring more assets to the merger with twice as many employees as Medlantic, 59 percent more hospital beds, 16 percent more revenue, and 132 percent more profit during 1997. Although Helix owned four Baltimore hospitals, none could compare with the range, scale, and services of Medlantic's Washington Hospital Center.[21]

Aided by a consultant, Merson and McDaniel constructed what they called—like so many hospital merger-makers[22]—a merger of equals, though Merson recognized that Helix would benefit more from the union than would Medlantic.[17,21] The new company would be called MedStar Health. Its board would have eighteen members, nine each from the Helix and Medlantic boards. At least six of the members would be physicians. The chairwoman of the Helix board would chair the new board.[23] More physicians would be added to the boards of the subsidiary hospitals.[17]

The founders[24] saw their merger involving two systems, Helix and Medlantic, in two markets with two different payment arrangements, Maryland remaining the only state with regulated hospital rates.[25] Their general methods of operating would need to be resolved, Helix's administration being more centralized than Medlantic's.[26]

When the Georgetown University Hospital was added in 2000, MedStar would include three hospitals in Washington—the Hospital Center, Georgetown, and the National Rehabilitation Hospital—and four in Baltimore.

Significant features of the merger would include:[21,24]

- *Creation of the largest medical system* in the Baltimore-Washington corridor, larger than the systems created by Johns Hopkins Medicine, the University of Maryland Medical System, or the other university hospitals in Washington.
- *More effective ability to compete for managed care contracts* with the health insurance companies because of its size.
- *Avoidance of expensive marketing campaigns* and what *The Washington Post* called a "medical arms race" as Medlantic and Helix expanded into each other's territories. "The Baltimore-Washington corridor," McDaniel told the *Post,* "from a business perspective and a health care delivery standpoint, has become, in effect, one marketplace."[21]
- *Few layoffs* since few of the services that Helix or Medlantic supplied overlapped with those of the other. As Merson told the *Baltimore Sun,* "Part of our agenda over time is to seek economic efficiencies

where we can, but we're not going to do it by focusing on work-force reductions."[23]

- *A decentralized structure,* since as John McDaniel says, "Health care is local."[24] MedStar would retain, however, the final decision on all significant financial and managerial issues. Searches for senior positions would be conducted locally, but the corporation would preserve the power to approve or reject those nominated.

On May 7, 1998, the boards of Helix and Medlantic approved the merger.[23] The new company would have 21,000 employees, 7 hospitals, 2,300 registered acute-care beds, 100,000 patient admissions annually, 5 nursing homes, 4,500 affiliated doctors, a medical equipment company, a radiology oncology company, and home care and rehabilitation centers. Annual revenue of the new company and its assets would each equal $1.4 billion.[23,27]

Officers

The board of the new corporation—composed of an equal number of trustees from Helix and Medlantic—elected John McDaniel chief executive officer and Kenneth Samet chief operating officer. Why was McDaniel rather than Merson chosen to head the company?[17]

- McDaniel had held executive positions in both Baltimore and Washington and thus had worked in both regulated and unregulated environments.
- McDaniel enjoyed the full support of his board, whereas Merson had been recast as CEO recently, and there was concern that his troubles with Union Memorial Hospital would resurface.
- McDaniel had greater experience in governmental and charitable activities in both communities than Merson had in either.
- Merson believed that he would bring the company his demonstrated abilities in planning, strategy, and coordinating administration, more suitable for the number two position.

The chief operating officer for the hospitals and the chief financial officer would report to the CEO, while other corporate and administrative functionaries reported to Merson, who would report to McDaniel.

The arrangement lasted for one year. "The model," Merson explains, "required very substantial sacrifices on the part of the other senior executives since we entered the merger with much duplication."[17] Worried that if they consolidated the positions immediately and believing that there was enough work for everyone, McDaniel and Merson decided to continue to employ all the executives from Helix and Medlantic. "We did not appreciate the amount of angst that adjusting to the new positions and reporting relationships would cause," said Merson. "The harmony that was needed did not come about."[17] The senior management group, Merson thought, was producing more friction by trying to divide McDaniel from him.[8]

Merson describes what followed. "We decided that it would not get better without a change in management. There was a short-term need for a more command and control, focused structure. John and I planned a reorganization that would give John more authority. I had to go to do this. It was inevitable."[17]

Merson left the company with four years left on his contract, providing that he did not take a job with a competing health care or insurance company in the region in which MedStar was operating. He was asked to, and agreed to, continue serving for three years on the planning and finance committees as a nonmember of the board.

The former CEO of Franklin Square Hospital and Helix Healthcare then became chairman of the restructured board of CareFirst, Blue Cross/Blue-Shield.[17,28,29] The giant insurer was recovering from a much-reported controversy with the state's legislature[30] and insurance commissioner[31] when it had attempted unsuccessfully to convert to a for-profit company. Franklin Square asked Merson to return for three months as interim CEO when the chief executive left. He also consults "in areas of improving hospital and health system governance, succession planning, executive compensation, and mergers and acquisitions."[32]

Washington Hospital Center

The centerpiece of MedStar's and earlier Medlantic's organization is the Washington Hospital Center, which opened in 1958 in North Washington by incorporating three older hospitals—Garfield, Episcopal, and Eye and

Ear.* The federal government provided the land, built the hospital, and briefly supported the costs of operating it.[33] In 1960 the government gave the deed and title for the forty-seven-acre campus to a not-for-profit corporation that would own and operate the Hospital Center. Subsequently, the corporation, named Medlantic in 1980, built the National Rehabilitation Hospital and merged with several other hospitals, each of which subsequently closed or was sold, and in the mid-1990s discussed with George Washington University the purchase of its hospital. The transaction never materialized.†

The Washington Hospital Center now occupies a forty-seven-acre campus in North Washington that it shares with three other medical facilities: the Department of Veterans Affairs Medical Center, the Children's National Medical Center, and the National Rehabilitation Hospital.[34]‡ With 900 beds and an average daily census of about 800, the Washington Hospital Center is 3 times the size of any other hospital in the district.[35] About 45,000 patients are admitted per year, and the doctors on the staff care for more than 350,000 outpatients. Most of the Hospital Center's 1,600 doctors and dentists practice privately in their own offices, many of which are located on the hospital's campus.

Financially, the Hospital Center has not always been the healthy institution that it earlier was and has recently become. By the beginning of the 1990s, the Hospital Center was losing money[36] and "had only four days of cash on hand," according to Kenneth Samet, who had started at Medlantic as John McDaniel's resident in 1982, became the hospital president in 1990, and is now (2008) MedStar's president and chief executive officer.[34] The reasons will sound familiar to all hospital directors: poor collection of bills, inadequate cost reporting, beds unfilled, large amounts of debt.[34,36] The hospital was also employing more than a hundred full-time physicians.[34]

The number of indigent patients at the Hospital Center discouraged many well-insured patients from coming there. Only the District of Columbia General Hospital gave care to more indigent patients than the Hospital

---

*The name MedStar derives from *Me*d*ical *S*hock/*T*rauma *A*cute *R*esuscitation unit, the name of a program for treating trauma patients established by the Washington Hospital Center in 1979.[33]

†For details about Medlantic's attempt to buy the George Washington University Hospital, see chapter 2.

‡President Abraham Lincoln's "Summer White House" was located here.[34]

Center.[37] After DC General closed in 2001, even more poorly insured patients came to the Washington Hospital Center's clinics and emergency department and for admission to its beds.* The Hospital Center's helicopter service, which feeds the district's largest emergency service, has grown into one of the busiest hospital-based transport services in the country.[35]

As admissions through the emergency department and to the medical and pediatric services grew, the finances began to look less favorable than in hospitals where the better-compensated surgical specialties predominated.[36] Concern about getting to the hospital through some of Washington's tougher districts convinced many potential patients to attend community hospitals in Maryland or Northern Virginia. More recently, however, the proportion of uninsured patients—about 5 percent received uncompensated care in 2005—decreased as the area surrounding the Hospital Center gentrified.[38]

The achievements of the Hospital Center and its current financial success owe much to its excellent and longtime reputation in cardiac services, where the cardiology patients formerly admitted to Georgetown are now treated. Well-respected surgeons and an active cardiac catheterization program† bring many patients to the hospital from the district and the suburban Maryland area. In successfully developing its cardiac services, the Hospital Center did just what Georgetown could not manage to do.[40]

Ken Samet invested in programs he saw as winners rather than spreading capital to all the specialties. "Not enough resources," he said. "If you do, everything is average."[34] He built new laboratories and operating rooms and bought the equipment that a leading center providing cardiac services required. Samet catered to the needs of the volunteer physicians who dominated and still dominate[41] the institution, the opposite of Georgetown's practice of building up its full-time staff and disfavoring privately practicing doctors.[40] "He changed the Hospital Center from a small community hospital—very provincial at the time—into a big and famous place," remembers Kenneth Kent, a leading cardiologist there.[40]

However, even the Hospital Center has been affected by the growing

---

* As a level 1 trauma center, the hospital is charged to provide the highest level of definitive and comprehensive care for patients with complex injuries. This adds to the number of uninsured patients the hospital must care for.[36]

† One of the three busiest in the country, according to Dr. Martin Leon, who led the lab in the 1990s.[39] Leon now works at the Presbyterian branch of New York–Presbyterian Hospital.

ability of medical cardiologists to carry out in their laboratories much of the work the surgeons had previously performed with the coronary artery bypass graft (CABG) operation. The number of surgical procedures dropped from about 3,200 cases in 1999 to about 2,000 six years later. Since cardiac surgery is among a hospital's most profitable activities—significantly more lucrative than the work done by cardiologists that may be equally effective medically—and with insurers paying less for the procedures, the financial implications were and continue to be serious.[40]

The Washington Hospital Center had long had an affiliation with the George Washington University School of Medicine. Hospital Center doctors held clinical professorial appointments at GW, and George Washington medical students took some of their clinical courses there. The affiliation began to fail as the two hospitals competed more intensively for patients, the financial climate worsened, and rivalry for house officers and fellows increased. GW leaders feared that rotating students though the Hospital Center might convince some to take their postgraduate training there rather than at George Washington. Opportunities for Hospital Center doctors to serve on committees at the medical school stopped. That the Hospital Center's census was several times larger than that at the George Washington University Hospital added to the angst.[42] So the Hospital Center began to look elsewhere for a more successful affiliation with a medical school.

Buying Georgetown

After integrating the Washington Hospital Center and the National Rehabilitation Hospital and then merging Medlantic with Helix, the leaders of MedStar considered where they could develop further. Trying to buy additional hospitals in the region would be difficult and, when MedStar tried, it did not succeed. Northern Virginia was dominated by Inova Health System and its successful Fairfax Hospital. In Washington, the thriving and fiercely independent Sibley Hospital seemed to be the only hospital suitable for acquisition, but Sibley was not interested in being acquired by anyone.[36] And then there was Georgetown University Hospital.

John McDaniel wanted MedStar to own a university hospital. Though he had failed with George Washington, the Georgetown University Hospital was available and in need of a dramatic solution to relieve the university of the financial problems the medical center was causing. MedStar had several reasons to look with favor on acquiring Georgetown.[24,36,40,43-51]

Competition. To a significant degree, merging with Georgetown would be defensive for MedStar, which feared the inevitable competition with the Washington Hospital Center, particularly for its high-intensity programs. McDaniel had long opposed the entry of for-profit hospitals into the Washington area, and the possibility that Georgetown might sell to such a company alarmed him. He feared that for-profits—and one now existed in the district at George Washington—would attract some of MedStar's well-insured and wealthier patients.

Administration. Washington Hospital Center's administrative experience and skills could be applied at Georgetown to improve its managerial and organizational operations and reduce its losses.

Location. Because Georgetown was on the west side of town and the Hospital Center was located more centrally, direct competition for patients would be less than if they were closer together. Furthermore, the Washington Hospital Center was often full and beds were unavailable for the admission of sick patients. MedStar hoped it could off-load some of its surplus to the Georgetown hospital, which was not filled.

Managed care. Owning two general hospitals in the district, MedStar would be able to negotiate better rates for managed care contracts. Before the merger, Georgetown's contracts paid poorly because the medical center, in one executive's words, "gave in on so many things."[43] When Georgetown objected to the low rates the managed care companies would pay, they would simply say, "Take it or leave it."[45]

Recruiting. Being able to give Georgetown faculty appointments would help MedStar convince high-quality clinicians and investigators to work at the Washington Hospital Center as well as at the university.

Training. Washington Hospital Center had long had difficulty recruiting qualified U.S. medical graduates to some of its internships, residencies, and fellowship training programs. Merger with Georgetown, it was hoped, would alleviate this problem.

Research. Through the collaboration with Georgetown, the research programs at the Hospital Center could flourish.

Prestige. Although MedStar, through its Washington Hospital Center, had programs such as cardiac surgery that were well known and respected inside and outside the district, it did not have the distinction associated with an intimate relationship with a university and its medical school. MedStar wanted to have, and be recognized as having, an academic medical center.

Local observers said:

- "MedStar bought it for the Georgetown seal. The Georgetown logo had value for them."
- "The academic panache that comes with owning an academic hospital would help fundraising."
- "They needed an academic partner to compete better with Hopkins."
- "Washington Hospital Center was the blue-collar guy who wanted to get into the country club."

Some of John McDaniel's colleagues did not favor acquiring Georgetown as much as he did. Kenneth Samet, MedStar's chief operating officer and McDaniel's closest associate, felt that owning a medical school hospital was not necessary to successfully deliver health care.[52] Samet and Michael O'Boyle, the chief financial officer at the time, also feared that Georgetown's sizeable losses would affect MedStar's financial status. The Georgetown University Hospital was losing money, and its accumulated deficits, carried by the university that owned it, exceeded $100 million. The hospital's average cash flow was negative, making the hospital a distressed asset. As O'Boyle observed, "We couldn't find much value in the hospital, though the university tried to make it appear more valuable than it was. The university equated value of the enterprise to the amount of debt they were carrying on the facility, and we couldn't support this."[36]

McDaniel's eagerness for the Georgetown imprimatur together with some effective bargaining by the Georgetown trustees led MedStar to pay a total of $95 million for the purchase. Critics saw compensating Georgetown even $25 million, for whatever strategic value the hospital might offer MedStar, was "a stretch."

"If his colleagues hadn't restrained him," one observer commented, "McDaniel might have paid even more." No other not-for-profit firm seemed to want the hospital,[44] and many at the university suspected that MedStar could have bought it for a token amount. Why should the purchaser assume responsibility for the accumulated losses that the university was carrying? they wondered.

"The Georgetown negotiators bluffed their way into the settlement," Dr. Paul Corso, the senior cardiac surgeon at the Hospital Center and a MedStar trustee, said.[53] Ned Cassem, the Jesuit psychiatrist on the Georgetown board at the time, saw "smirks" on the faces of several of his colleagues over how much MedStar was agreeing to pay. "They couldn't see where the value was."[54] Winston Churchill, however, one of the Georgetown trustees intimately involved in the sale, says that the amount the university received for the sale was "a fair price."[55]

What MedStar paid to the university strongly affected the parent company's balance sheet by reducing funds available for improvements needed at the Georgetown Hospital and at the other MedStar hospitals and Med-Star's bond rating.[34,36,53] Some of the executives of the Baltimore hospitals feared that the purchase would decrease the support they might otherwise receive for favorite projects.[35,36] Would some of the doctors at the Hospital Center move to Georgetown, thereby weakening the flagship?[36] Might MedStar have been able to convert the Georgetown University Hospital's operating losses into a surplus more quickly if it hadn't paid the university so much to acquire the hospital?

McDaniel, supported by William Thomas, MedStar's executive vice president for medical affairs,[56] and the MedStar trustees, prevailed, and Med-Star acquired its own university hospital. McDaniel became a Georgetown trustee, and John DeGioia, soon to be Georgetown's president, joined the MedStar board.[36]

MedStar System

By 2006, MedStar had become what John McDaniel describes as "a multi-institutional, not-for-profit health care organization serving Washington, D.C., Maryland, Virginia, and the mid-Atlantic region . . . an integrated system of 25 hospitals and health care businesses. MedStar is the third largest employer in the region, with more than 23,000 employees and 4,000 affiliated physicians, serving more than half-a-million patients each year."[24] MedStar has 15 percent of the hospital business in the Baltimore-Washington corridor. Johns Hopkins has two-thirds as much as MedStar, and the University of Maryland one-half.[56]

MedStar delegates much of its day-to-day administration to the executives at the constituent hospitals. They develop budgets, elaborate strategic planning, recruit doctors and administrators, and then present their advice to the central administration for approval or modification. Each of the hospitals is also responsible for relations with doctors, philanthropy, community support, and mission.[26]

The executives at corporate headquarters in Columbia, Maryland, perform most of the back-office financial functions for each of the hospitals, including payroll; accounts payable and receivable; financial policies, procedures, and reports; targets for budgets; general accounting; and treasury functions, including investments, cash, and debt. Billing is performed in a centralized billing office for all the hospitals except the Hospital Center and Union Memorial Hospital.[26] "There are logistical issues that make further centralization difficult at this time," explains John Marzano, MedStar's corporate director for communications.[57]

Other functions also centralized at corporate headquarters include purchasing, legal, compliance and audit, and information technology. Corporate negotiates managed care contracts for all the hospitals. Both the hospitals and the corporate headquarters develop government relationships, long-range planning, and efficiencies in a matrix arrangement.

As the union with Georgetown progressed, much discussion was devoted to how much the hospital's administrative functions should be centralized. "Let's do what works best financially," advised MedStar's current chief financial officer, Mike Curran. "That makes the best business sense."[26] The other MedStar executives agreed that MedStar could administer more effectively than Georgetown. "It was important," Marzano adds, "to move away from university-based processes and into hospital-based processes."[57]

Does MedStar's partially centralized structure inhibit the hiring of first-rate executives at the local hospitals? "We've not seen this," says Curran. "It's a good learning experience early in their careers, and we provide plenty of opportunities for advancement at the hospitals or at corporate."[26]*

The MedStar board includes the top executives of the corporation, the president of Georgetown University,† several leading physicians from the system's hospitals, and the usual group of influential lawyers and executives

---

*The ultimate examples of this are John McDaniel, MedStar's chief executive officer, and Kenneth Samet, MedStar's president and chief operating officer until 2008. Both were presidents of the Washington Hospital Center earlier in their careers.

†In recognition of MedStar's owning the Georgetown University Hospital and the Georgetown Physician Group.

who populate such boards. Each of the constituent hospitals retains its own board, which works with the local executives on quality assurance, certification of the professional staff, community relations, and fundraising.[34] Even though these trustees do not have the ultimate authority that the MedStar board possesses, many of the local trustees prefer to support their own hospitals rather than work for the more removed senior board, which bears responsibility for a company with $2.5 billion in assets. "The hospital boards must relate to their local communities," explains Ken Samet.[34] The corporate rules do not allow trustees to serve simultaneously on a local hospital board and on the MedStar board.[34]

Medical Affairs

Dr. William Thomas is the executive vice president for medical affairs and the chief medical officer for the MedStar Health system.* His office is at the corporate headquarters in Columbia, Maryland. Thomas has overall responsibility for graduate and continuing medical education, affiliation agreements, insurance, risk management, and quality assurance throughout the MedStar Health system. The vice presidents for medical affairs (chief medical officers) at each of MedStar's seven hospitals and its home health division deal with the more day-to-day activities in these areas. Thomas chairs the administration of MedStar's off-shore malpractice insurance for the hospitals and physicians.[2]

With the help of MedStar's centralized legal staff, each of the hospitals and services develops its own standards for disciplinary issues. "It's extremely valuable to the vice presidents for medical affairs in the small hospitals to be able to draw on the experiences in other parts of the company in this work," says Thomas.[2] Its centralized system has allowed MedStar to improve the oversight of the graduate medical education programs and manage more effectively the reimbursement of the trainees. Thomas explains: "Such matters are no longer at the whim of individuals in the different departments."[2]

---

*Thomas (B.S., Duke; M.D., Connecticut) is a general internist who was chairman of the department of medicine, vice president for medical affairs, and director of medical education at Franklin Square Hospital—where he met Michael Merson—and from 1994 to 1998 chairman of the board of directors and senior vice president for medical affairs at Helix before taking his current position at MedStar.

MedStar Research Institute

Thomas also helps to direct research within the system through the Med-Star Research Institute. The institute, which has its own board of directors that reports to the MedStar corporate board, supervises all research performed in each unit of MedStar except at the Georgetown University Hospital.[58]

In the spring of 2006, the annual revenue of the MedStar Research Institute was about $50 million, half in grants and contracts from the federal government and the other half from pharmaceutical and devices companies and foundations.[58] Most is not from the National Institutes of Health (NIH).* The cardiology division accounts for 24 percent of this budget.[46] Doctors who spend more than about 50 percent in research tend to be employed in the research institute, as do all Ph.D.s.[42] Clinicians doing clinical research are MedStar hospital employees, and most have faculty appointments at Georgetown.

That some investigators at the Washington Hospital Center "continue to think that the Georgetown people look down on them and feel threatened by them" is a problem, says Barbara Howard, the former president of the Research Institute. "It's not an easy issue to fix, but I think it's getting better."[58]

A similar spirit exists among the Georgetown and Hospital Center physicians, says Mark Smith, the chairman of emergency medicine at both institutions. "It's caused by a 'cultural divide.'[61] The Hospital Center staff thinks the Georgetown docs like to work 9 to 3 and want their residents to do the work. Georgetown sees the doctors at the Hospital Center as plumbers, not as good docs."[35] The Hospital Center takes care of more African American patients than Georgetown, whose clientele is predominately white. "It's an inner-city versus a more privileged institution difference," says Smith.[35]

As for research, "I am trying to encourage collaboration and with some success," says Dr. Robert Ratner, the Research Institute's vice president for scientific affairs, "and move clinical research forward within the MedStar health system."[62] An endocrinologist, Ratner spent the first ten years of his

---

*The institute received $16,884,528 for 11 grants from the NIH in 2005, placing it 41st among 273 research institutes.[59] The Georgetown medical school received $58,907,122.[60]

career after finishing training at George Washington. In 1992 he left because "I felt the president and the dean were providing disincentives to performing research. About 25 to 33 percent of the clinical faculty left when I did."[62] He moved to the Washington Hospital Center as director of the section of diabetes, metabolism, and nutrition and the clinical research center. Because the Hospital Center was then affiliated with the university, he continued his academic appointment at GW until 2001. Ratner's current academic appointment is professor of medicine at Georgetown.

One of the MedStar's most renowned investigators is Dr. Stephen Epstein, who directs the Cardiovascular Research Institute (CRI),* which is based at the Washington Hospital Center. Epstein came to MedStar in 1998 from the National Heart, Lung, and Blood Institute of the NIH, where he had been chief of the cardiology branch for thirty years. "One of the wisest decisions of my professional life," Epstein describes his move to the MedStar Research Institute.[63] Epstein's work concentrates on translational research, based on vascular biology, some now done in collaboration with scientists at Georgetown. MedStar's CRI has a hundred employees, forty of whom are professional investigators holding the degrees of M.D. or Ph.D.[64]

New Challenges

In the fiscal year ending June 30, 2005, MedStar made $17 million in operations. Excess of revenues over expenses ("bottom bottom" line) was $40 million.[46] By 2006, each of the MedStar hospitals was profitable on operations. MedStar plans to invest $140 million of its capital in various improvements during fiscal year 2007.[53] Despite this good news, however, MedStar's executives, like most leaders in the hospital business, continue to worry about where the capital needed to renovate and improve hospital buildings, many of which are more than thirty years old, will come from.

MedStar has added no more hospitals to its collection since buying Georgetown in 2000. The company needed time to "digest" its most recent purchase.[65] By 2006, however, with the Georgetown University Hospital making a surplus, the executives could look more confidently toward what they should do next. Most of the current plans involve improving what they have rather than acquiring more hospitals.

*Successor to the Cardiovascular Research Foundation.

The company is urging the doctors to accept electronic medical records, establish service lines among the hospitals—initially in neurosciences and cardiovascular and vascular surgery—control malpractice rates, improve safety and quality of services, and develop protocols for delivery of care. MedStar also wants to help the physicians run their practices more efficiently.

Should MedStar increase the number of full-time physicians it employs? As the result of a conscious effort to discourage private practice at Georgetown, almost all its doctors there are full-time members of the MedStar-owned practice plan. At the Washington Hospital Center—which made its reputation on the private practice model[65]—and in all of the Baltimore hospitals, most of the doctors are in private practice.

"We're being pushed into it," believes Christine Swearingen, senior vice president for corporate strategy and business development at MedStar. "We need better coverage of our emergency department and in many subspecialties. The privates can't do it." For full-time employees, MedStar can use its size to leverage the insurance companies for lower malpractice rates than private practitioners can obtain. "We need to partner more with our doctors considering the pressure they're under," Swearingen said.[65]

In 2006, the department of medicine had about 70 full-time physicians, more than in any other department. The cardiology division had 20, the most in the department. Each of the other divisions had between 4 and 7.* Unlike at most major teaching hospitals, MedStar charges no tax on the earnings of the full-time doctors. Leonard Wartofsky, the chairman of medicine at the Hospital Center, suspects that full-time employment is becoming more attractive even to the doctors who have been wedded to private practice in the past. "Some are looking for stable jobs."[42]†

With MedStar's hospitals located in regions where the population was not growing, the company has to look outside itself. There are few hospitals that the company could acquire even if it wanted to, and MedStar is not positioned to grow beyond its region.[36] Inova owns Northern Virginia, and few of the hospitals in Washington and Baltimore potentially attractive to

---

*Nuclear medicine is a division of the department of medicine at the Hospital Center. All of its members are full-time.

†Departments need full-time doctors to be eligible for approved training programs. Each of the surgeons in the large and historically very successful cardiac surgical program practices privately, many in groups. Accordingly, despite the many patients and variety of procedures, the Hospital Center trains no fellows in this subspecialty.[42]

MedStar are free-standing. So MedStar is looking toward useful affiliations. The company is talking to the officers of a regional hospital that wants help developing a cardiac program. "Unless we link to them, we could lose the business they now send to us," explains Christine Swearingen.[65]

The tenure of John McDaniel, CEO of Medlantic since 1982 and of Med-Star since its creation in 1998, has occupied the attention of those who speculate about such matters. Kenneth Samet, currently the MedStar president, is thought to be the leading candidate to succeed him as CEO. As knowledge of his and MedStar's successes has spread, Samet has become a candidate for, and has been offered, the CEO position at several leading teaching hospitals and multi-institutional systems. So far, he has not moved. McDaniel and the board appreciate his value—"Ken Samet's the brains behind the operation," one of the leading cardiologists in Washington has said[40]—have put him on the MedStar board, and made it financially worth his while not to leave.

Samet's patience has borne fruit. At the beginning of 2007, John Mc-Daniel announced that he would resign the CEO position at the end of the year and that Kenneth Samet would succeed him. "This will ensure a continuity of leadership for MedStar Health well into the future," McDaniel predicted.[66]

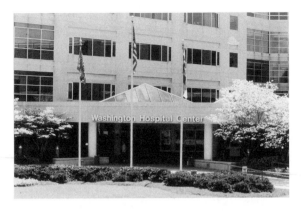

Washington Hospital Center, MedStar's flagship and the District of Columbia's largest hospital. *Courtesy of MedStar Health*

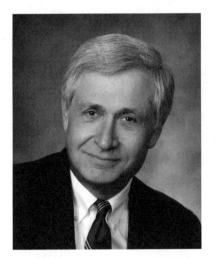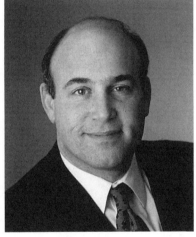

John McDaniel (*left*), CEO of MedStar Health and the force behind acquiring the Georgetown University Hospital and the medical school's practice plan for full-time faculty. Kenneth Samet (*right*), MedStar's president and chief operating officer and McDaniel's successor in 2008. In his previous position as president of the Washington Hospital Center, Samet was instrumental in developing it into a leading provider of health care in the city. *Courtesy of MedStar Health*

CHAPTER TEN

Conclusions

Selling the Hospitals

George Washington and Georgetown had to sell their hospitals.* Both
had lost large amounts of money for several years, and neither university
could reverse the losses. The principal external stimulus for the losses was
decreased compensation for hospital and professional care, produced by
managed care and the Balanced Budget Act of 1997, which was inadequate
to cover the rising costs of providing care. Neither institution could obtain
assistance from the District of Columbia or federal government. Neither
government had supported the hospitals at Georgetown and George Washington for decades nor seemed inclined to do so when they needed help.

A major internal force causing the losses in both medical centers was
the absence of the administrative and financial skills needed to manage
the medical centers in a time of falling revenues and increasing expenses.
George Washington was burdened with an outdated, long undercapitalized

---

*And, in so doing, joined the majority of universities in which the governance of medical schools
and teaching hospitals is separate.[1]

hospital that would require more money to renovate or replace than the university was prepared to spend or borrow. Though not showing its wear as obviously, the Georgetown University Hospital also needed investment in facilities and equipment.

Eventually, the trustees and officers of the two universities despaired of repairing their finances and sold the hospitals to whoever would buy them and guarantee the continuation of the academic missions of the two medical schools. By the time the two hospitals were sold, the universities had few realistic alternatives to the companies that were chosen.

George Washington sold to a national, for-profit, hospital-owning corporation, a resolution chosen by few other medical schools.[2]* There seems little question, however, that the decision has proven to be wise for the university. Ten years after the sale, GW has a fine new teaching hospital, financed, built, and managed by a company that specializes in constructing and running hospitals effectively and economically unlike the university, which had demonstrated its inability to do either.

Georgetown sold to a local not-for-profit entity, whose CEO was eager to own a university teaching hospital. Like George Washington, Georgetown had few alternatives. Its Jesuit nature made selling to a for-profit corporation undesirable. The other leading not-for-profit company in the area presented terms that could not compare with what MedStar was prepared to offer. In addition to the cost of buying the hospital and practice plan, the purchaser would also have to invest in improving the hospital structure and function and absorb losses until the hospital began to produce surpluses.

Like at GW, most at Georgetown agree that the sale was wise. Its hospital is now well managed, its facilities upgraded, and its financial condition improved, none of which the university could have accomplished by itself.

Selling the Practice Plans

Both George Washington and Georgetown cast off their practice plans for full-time faculty. George Washington created an independent corporation called Medical Faculty Associates, Inc. (MFA) for its doctors, and Georgetown sold theirs to the company that bought the hospital. Money

*See appendix A.

was an important reason in both cases. George Washington's plan was in deficit, and, although Georgetown's was said to be solvent, the university feared that the plan would lose money in the future. At Georgetown, MedStar, which bought the hospital, insisted on acquiring the plan to assure that the doctors would contribute to the recovery of the hospital by practicing more effectively and efficiently than when they were employed by the university.

Conversion from university employment was painful, according to members of the clinical faculty at Georgetown. Less generous medical coverage and pensions, no more university tenure, and loss of tuition benefits and of status as university employees hurt. Although conversion certainly caused distress, the passage of seven years has mellowed the faculty's disappointment and anger, in some cases, about the change. The experience at both medical schools should warn other institutions considering such a change that the process will not be free from trouble.

As for finances, the conversions have been salutary. MFA has repaired its deficit, a result attributed in part to removing the university with its inadequate administrative procedures from operating the plan and transferring it to the doctors themselves to run. At Georgetown, the finances of the practice plan are melded into those of the hospital, and two together are now producing a surplus.

The most important academic effect at both medical schools has been the loss of control of the full-time clinical faculty by the medical schools. Although at GW the dean is a member of MFA's board of trustees, his ability to influence how the doctors spend their time and the money they generate from practicing medicine is limited. In particular, he cannot effectively stimulate them to perform research since their compensation is predicated on the success of their practices and the efficient operation of the enterprise.

MFA itself invests little in the research infrastructure needed for successful research programs to grow nor does it support the salaries of its members to perform unfunded research or invest in recruiting established or young, as yet unfunded, clinical faculty who desire research careers. The MFA leaders direct any surpluses that the practice generates to improving how the practice operates and to paying their salaries and benefits, not unexpectedly since MFA is an independent, multi-specialty group practice that contracts with the George Washington medical school to teach its students and trainees.

Unlike at George Washington, where the clinicians run their practice corporation, at Georgetown MedStar is the doctors' boss. They now work for an organization that is administering the Georgetown clinical establishment much more efficiently and financially successfully than did the university. The emphasis on practice, however, is no different from what their contemporaries face at George Washington. Also like with MFA, MedStar recruits few doctors or financially supports current clinical faculty to be investigators unless they can bring with them grants to defray their salaries and the expenses associated with their studies. MedStar insists that any surpluses the clinical departments develop be spent for clinical and not academic purposes. The leader of the school of medicine must rely on whatever influence he can exert on the management at MedStar to support research productivity from most of the clinical faculty.

Money for Clinical Teaching

The agreement establishing the practice corporation at George Washington prescribed that the school pay the physician group to supply clinical instruction to the medical students. The current figure of $11.6 million[3] is based on "historical data," according to GW medical center officials.[4]

Georgetown leaders went through a complex numerical exercise, helped by a consultant and internal committees, to develop a formula that Med-Star and the medical school could accept for the clinical instruction of Georgetown medical students. Based on former subsidies to the departments, they reached the figure of $9 million, to be allocated annually from tuition income to MedStar for distribution among the clinical departments and the doctors.[5,6]

Unlike at George Washington and Georgetown, most medical schools do not know what they spend for the clinical instruction of their medical students. This was what I learned from e-mailing executive vice presidents, deans, chief financial officers, and members of their staffs at 117 medical schools. Officials from 90 schools responded.[4,5,7-103]

Seventeen schools had specific data. In table 1, the average amounts per student are compared for two classes in the third and fourth years.*

---

* $ divided by students per class times 2.

Table 1. *Amounts Spent for Clinical Instruction*

School	$ (millions) for clinical teaching	Students per class	$ (thousands) per student in third and fourth years
Arizona[52]	12.5	110	57
Florida, Gainesville[98]	6.6	108	31
George Washington[3,93]	11.6	164	35
Georgetown[5]	9	190	23
Georgia, Medical College of[71]	15.6	190	41
Indiana[62]	20	280	35
Loma Linda[99]	5.8	175	17
Missouri, Kansas City[27]	5	100	25
Penn State, Hershey (2005–6)[43]	4.5	152	15
Pennsylvania[74]	3.8	150	17
Pittsburgh[64]	14.2	145	48
South Dakota [55]	3.4	50	34
Texas A&M[21]	4.85	85	28
Texas, Medical Branch, Galveston[65]	13	200	23
Vermont[33]	5.1	110	23
Virginia[38]	13	142	45
Wisconsin–Madison[104]	12	150	40

When asking for comparable data elsewhere, I received the following answers, which are representative of the responses from most of the schools:

- "As you know, tracking the exact cost of educating a medical student is difficult."
- "I don't know precisely."
- "There's no way of calculating the amount."
- "This seemingly simple question is too hard to answer, because money flows in many different ways."
- "We don't quantify in the way you are looking for, and I'd be surprised if anyone has a true and accurate number."
- "Now that is an impossible question."

Troubles Recruiting

The changes at both medical schools appear to have impeded recruiting strong leadership from other medical schools in the clinical departments and, in Georgetown's case, in basic science as well.

At George Washington, only two clinicians—in pediatrics and urology—have been brought from other medical schools to chair clinical departments. The pediatrics recruitment was conducted by the Washington Children's Hospital, an independent institution with which GW is affiliated. At the main campus, the chairman of urology came from Johns Hopkins. All other clinical chairs have been filled by internal appointments. Because of the expense recruiting the new chairman of urology, Medical Faculty Associates decided in 2006 not to recruit other clinical chairmen from outside GW.

Recruitment of clinicians at Georgetown rests with MedStar, and as of 2006, most of the appointments were based on clinical work. MedStar does not support clinical research at Georgetown, and with the clinical chairmen as well as all the clinicians being MedStar employees, the school can exercise little direct influence on how these departments develop academically. Since the sale, only the chairman of surgery has been recruited from elsewhere, George Washington in his case. Other chairmen have been appointed from within the institution usually following failed national searches or without such searches being conducted at all.

Does transferring ownership of the practice plans explain these events? The financial problems at each institution that led to the sale of the hospitals and the separation from their practice plans certainly contribute to difficulty recruiting. However, the impetus for developing academic programs traditionally originates at the medical school, where the chairmen respond to the dean's policy directives. Neither George Washington nor Georgetown can now provide that stimulus because of the structural independence of the practices from the medical schools.

At George Washington someday, a new executive vice president will be needed. Will a first-rate clinical academic want to lead a medical school without a practice plan and where the leading mission of the university hospital is other than serving the school's academic mission? Universal, despite its many contributions in building a new hospital and operating it efficiently, is a for-profit company ultimately responsible to its stockholders.

Georgetown has solved its leadership problem by appointing a distinguished neuroscientist, Dr. Howard Federoff of the University of Rochester, as its new dean and executive vice president. He has the stature and experience to develop strong basic science departments so long as the university is prepared to fund the effort. How to bring the company that controls the clinical enterprise into closer harmony with the medical school's academic mission is arguably his greatest challenge. Though MedStar is a not-for-profit company, its preeminent hospital is not the university hospital. The company's executives and the president of the Georgetown University Hospital, until she was appointed to the job, have never worked at primary university teaching hospitals. They run a well-managed, surplus-producing company, but their dedication to the academic mission of the medical school has not been, as of the winter of 2006–7, their primary concern.

Research

The leaders at both schools see their foremost mission to train students to become doctors and provide some of them with postgraduate training as residents and fellows in the hospitals and clinics associated with the schools. As best one call tell, both schools do these jobs well. Most of their graduates pass the qualifying examinations, some with excellent scores. They gain internships at competitive teaching hospitals and then pass the certifying examinations that follow this phase of training.

How well the average George Washington or Georgetown graduate functions in practice, when compared with those from other medical schools, is impossible to gauge. There are few comparative criteria to judge such performances once training with its examinations has been successfully completed. Given these records, it is reasonable to assume that most of the teachers at these schools fulfill what is expected of them, but comparing teaching ability among different schools is difficult.

The most measurable accomplishment of medical schools is research. There are several schedules that compare this ability, but the most frequently cited is the record of grants, contracts, and fellowships funded by the National Institutes of Health (NIH). On the schedule for 2005, the two schools studied for this book do not rank high, George Washington at 92nd (from 121 schools with NIH support) and Georgetown at 60th.

These records are not new. Georgetown has had better days, ranking in the 40s thirty years ago. GW's NIH rank has consistently been low. Why haven't these schools flourished in research?

Except in the early years of the John Griffith administration at Georgetown, university administrations at both George Washington and Georgetown have not emphasized making their medical schools research-intensive. Furthermore, neither school has the endowment and other sources of money needed to build a research enterprise without support from their teaching hospitals, practice plans, and universities. Laboratory space at both schools may once have been a limiting factor but it has not been so for several decades.

The relevant question for this study is not so much why these schools have the record in research that they have, but how the sales of the hospitals and practice plans have affected this part of the schools' mission. One would have to conclude that they have not helped and may have hurt.

Investor-Owned Companies and Teaching Hospitals*

Zeal among the executives of for-profit hospital-owned companies to own university teaching hospitals seems to have disappeared. When buying these hospitals was in vogue, the companies considered such purchases to constitute "strategic product lines."[105] The companies knew that they could operate the hospitals more efficiently, effectively, and financially successfully than could the universities.

What they did not recognize when they made these purchases was that the universities and their medical schools would expect the hospital owners to provide significant and continuing support for their educational and other academic programs. These demands are problems that such companies do not have to deal with in their community hospitals.[105] And then there is the necessity of working with faculty members whose professional aims differ from those of the privately practicing doctors who admit patients to the companies' community hospitals. As a result of these pressures, among others, university hospitals cannot generate the amount of profit that the companies expect from their holdings.†

Consequently, investor-owned companies have lost their enthusiasm for buying hospitals in academic medical centers. Alan Miller, the president and CEO of Universal, which bought the George Washington University Hospital, specifically told me this for his company.[106] Phillip Schaengold, who led the GW hospital for Universal and worked for Tenet in senior corporate

---

*See appendix A.

†Generally, investor-owned companies expect their hospitals to generate earnings of about 15 percent on operations before interest, taxes, and depreciation (EBITD.)[105] Operating margins of 3 to 5 percent are considered quite acceptable at not-for-profit university hospitals which, of course, do not have to pay taxes. While Phillip Schaengold was working for Tenet from 2000 to 2004, "every Tenet academic medical center had a positive operating margin."[105]

positions in St. Louis and Philadelphia, agrees. "I doubt that investor-owned hospital corporations will buy any more university hospitals."[107]

The Future of George Washington Medicine

The George Washington and Georgetown medical schools are more similar than different. Each is predominately a clinical school, emphasizing education and clinical care. Each depends financially on charging high tuitions to its students and admitting large classes. Neither owns its hospital or practice plan. Each is weak in research. Both are located in the same city, a factor of not inconsequential importance.

At GW, the development most likely to affect the immediate and long-range future of the medical enterprise is the election of Steven Knapp as the new president of the university. Knapp, provost of Johns Hopkins University when chosen, has worked for more than a decade at an institution renowned for its outstanding school of medicine. Although not directly responsible for the medical school in the job he is leaving, Knapp has seen how much a successful medical program can contribute to the academic reputation of a university. If he decides to emphasize the development of academic medicine at George Washington, Knapp will need wholehearted support from his trustees to change the less than enthusiastic policies of his predecessor.

GW medicine's greatest weakness is research, a perpetual problem throughout the school's history. The obstacles to creating a research-intensive medical school at George Washington are several: lack of money to invest in the recruitment of first-rate medical scientists, ownership of the teaching hospital by a for-profit company, the structure of the practice plan, and, of great importance, the absence, throughout its history, of what critics at the school call a "research culture." If the new president and his associates should decide to convert GW into a research-intensive medical school—a priority that some may consider neither essential nor even desirable—decades of investment and effort will be needed.

Though a good partner for the university so far, Universal Health Services, Inc., which owns the George Washington University Hospital, uses its resources, as a for-profit company, more to maximize shareholder value than to support the academic mission of the university. If the school decides to promote research, it would benefit if the hospital were owned by

an independent, not-for-profit 501(c)(3) company whose primary obligation could be specified to assist the medical school by investing part of its
surpluses in support of GW's academic mission.* Universal might well sell
to such an organization if the price were right. Until an independent administration could be developed, Universal might be retained to manage
the hospital under its new structure.[108] Reacquiring ownership of the hospital by the university is an option that would be received with little enthusiasm by those faculty, executives, and trustees who remember the history of
troubles under that form of governance.

Medical Faculty Associates (MFA), successor to the medical school's full-
time practice plan, has not advanced clinical research in the school. To
strengthen this activity will require adjusting the relationship between
MFA and the school.

The Future of Georgetown Medicine

Georgetown's unique relationship with MedStar offers opportunities
not available to George Washington. The school now has, in effect, two
principal teaching hospitals, the Georgetown University Hospital, a relatively small, increasingly subspecialized institution, and the Washington
Hospital Center, a much larger general hospital. Thus Georgetown can provide more doctors, beds, and outpatient offices to serve the school's educational mission—all directly under the control of its partner, MedStar—than
can George Washington.

Like at GW, research is not Georgetown medicine's strong suit although,
of the two, Georgetown has the more distinguished record. During the
early administration of dean John Griffith in the 1980s, Georgetown tried
to develop this aspect of its mission, but, because of developments discussed in chapter 6, the medical school could not achieve Griffith's goal.
Recently, a few distinguished clinical investigators have come to the medical center, with both the university and MedStar contributing financially to
their recruitment. However, appointing new scientists in the basic science
departments has been frozen because of lack of money.

Since most private medical schools need significant financial support

*Ownership of teaching hospitals by organizations that are independent of the universities, such
as not-for-profit 501(c)(3) corporations, are by far the most common form of governance in both private and state-owned universities.[1]

from their teaching hospitals and practice plans to fulfill their academic missions, research at Georgetown will not flourish unless MedStar helps more than it has. As of the winter of 2006–7, MedStar sent the medical school no money for academic development. It is no wonder that the medical school requires a sizeable subsidy from the university despite charging one of the highest tuitions of any U.S. medical school to students in classes that are among the largest in the private schools.*

With the appointment of neuroscientist Howard Federoff from the University of Rochester as its leader, a new day for medical research at Georgetown may have arrived. The combination of the university hospital and Washington Hospital Center provides a superb opportunity for training students and graduate physicians and for conducting clinical research. However, for the school to become a significant source of the quality of research with which Federoff is familiar, MedStar must help.

For this to happen, MedStar's trustees and executives must undertake the conversion of the company into a truly academic medical center. As a starter, MedStar should change its rule that permanent chairmen of the clinical departments must be employed by the company rather than the university, a policy that will inhibit the recruitment of leading academic physicians from other institutions.† MedStar could sell its community hospitals in Baltimore—which refer few patients to the Washington hospitals—and invest some of the proceeds in the academic work of the medical school.

In time, the nation's capital might be able to claim, for the first time, the presence of a nationally recognized, first-class academic medical center and medical school.

---

*I could not learn why Georgetown's medical school needs a subsidy from its university to balance its books while GW does not. One observer has suggested that GW's having fewer scientific faculty may explain the difference.[109]

† If this rule is changed, chairmen could, with the collaboration of the hospital president, appoint associate chairmen who are MedStar employees to supervise the clinical work.

APPENDIX A

Other Universities with Teaching Hospitals Owned by For-Profit Companies[1]

Creighton University[2,3]

In 1984, the Creighton Omaha Regional Health Care Corporation, the parent body of St. Joseph's Hospital and St. Joseph's Center for Mental Health, the principal teaching affiliates of Creighton's school of medicine, sold its facilities to American Medical International (AMI), Inc. In the year before the sale, most of the beds at St. Joseph's were occupied with patients and the hospital was producing annual surpluses of about $500,000, but the leaders of the hospitals and university had become concerned that the future might not be as financially agreeable. AMI seemed more likely to develop the capital to improve the hospital than could local management.

The sale brought several years of progress to the medical center. "AMI brought superior management to the operation of the hospitals and improved its financial performance," remembers Dr. Richard O'Brien, dean of Creighton's medical school from 1982 to 1992.[4]

In 1990, AMI's leadership changed through a leveraged buyout, and the new management challenged several provisions of the original contract guaranteeing support of academic programs.* Creighton filed suit against AMI and explored the purchase of St. Joseph's Hospital and the mental health center from the company. AMI countersued. The controversy was settled in 1995, the year that AMI merged with National Medical Enterprises into the newly named corporation Tenet Healthcare. Court-ordered mediation resulted in an agreement to create a limited liability corporation to own the hospitals; Creighton would purchase 26 percent and Tenet the remaining 74 percent. The Creighton-affiliated institutions were the first major teaching hospitals that Tenet, and the corporations from which it was formed, had acquired.

"Overall, we're content with the arrangement," says Dr. Cam Enarson,

---

*Though rejecting the budget, AMI, for public relations purposes, it was presumed, continued to support the medical school as it had in the past.[4]

vice president for health sciences and dean of the school of medicine since 2003. The dean praises the ownership feature that lets the medical school influence effectively those decisions that affect its academic interests. "The collaboration is satisfactory, despite challenges," one of which is Tenet's well-publicized national difficulties, which, Enarson says, "we follow with interest."[5]

University of Southern California

In May 1991, the University of Southern California (USC) School of Medicine acquired its first university hospital, which had been built and was owned by National Medical Enterprises (NME), a for-profit hospital-owning corporation. NME* paid all costs for building the hospital—$157 million—on land leased from the university, originally for thirty years, later extended to 2062.[6,7] The USC University Hospital, currently with 269 beds, was designed primarily as a surgical hospital.[7] It provides no emergency, pediatrics, or obstetrics services.

USC and NME proceeded to recruit leading surgeons to join the faculty and work at the hospital. Though each acquired USC academic appointments, they continued to practice privately. Most of the referrals come from community physicians rather than from members of the school's other clinical departments. Until the university hospital opened, the university had owned only small specialty hospitals and not a hospital suitable for private, better-insured adult patients who might come to its faculty for care. University of Southern California medical students receive most of their clinical training at the Los Angeles County Hospital, which is adjacent to the school.

When NME became Tenet Healthcare in the mid-1990s, the governance did not change and continued to be wholly vested in the company. Tenet and USC each appoint half of the members of the hospital board.

As business grew, the USC University Hospital became and remains (as of the fall of 2006) Tenet's most profitable university hospital. Having no emergency department—the site of admission for many indigent patients—accepting no Medicaid contracts,† providing complex, sophisticated, re-munerative medical services, and controlling all the ancillary procedures help to make the hospital the money-making machine it has become for its owner.

---

*The CEO of NME at the time was Richard Eamer, a USC graduate.
†Called Medical in California.

The company continued the practice of recruiting doctors with successful practices who agree to contribute a portion of their incomes to their departments and to the school of medicine from their 501(c)(3) corporations. The dean, however, lacks the power to discharge the university hospital service chiefs, and the faculty there continues to practice privately. Tenet strongly influences which clinicians the departments recruit.

By 2004, as Tenet's legal and financial problems grew, the hospital management abruptly terminated its agreements with the doctors. Using the Stark laws "as cover,"* according to a senior member of the faculty, Tenet reduced what it was paying to support new programs at the hospital and to the service chiefs for their administrative work. The recent developments "greatly distracted the doctors and staff. The place was starting to look more and more like a community hospital," he said.

Then in the summer of 2006, articles appeared in the *Los Angeles Times*[7] and the *Wall Street Journal*[9] revealing that USC was suing Tenet to sell its ownership and control of the Hospital to USC. "The suit effectively claims," wrote the *Journal*'s reporter, "that Tenet has starved the USC hospital of needed capital investment and that government investigations into the hospital operator have hurt the university's ability to recruit top-notch physicians." Marshall Grossman, the Los Angeles lawyer representing the university, said, "We are filing this suit to regain† ownership of that facility so that it is within the destiny and control of USC and no longer beholden to a badly damaged Tenet."[9]

USC faculty leaders were becoming convinced that Tenet was a less reliable partner than in the past. As one of them said, "We're dealing with different missions: academic medicine at the university, making money for the stockholders and executives at Tenet."‡

Tulane University

The union of George Washington and Universal was based on a similar model developed in 1995 by Tulane University and HCA, the for-profit, hospital-owning corporation formerly called Hospital Corporation of America.[1,10] Like GW and Universal, Tulane sold 80 percent of its university

---

*The Stark laws, named for Pete Stark, Democratic congressman from California, deal with conflicts of interest when doctors refer patients to hospitals in which they have financial interests.[8]

†The word *regain* should be *acquire*. USC has never owned the hospital.

‡I interviewed several doctors at USC about these developments, but none wanted to be identified, presumably because of the lawsuit.

hospital to HCA. The two parties created a corporation to own the hospital—HCA manages it—with an equal number of board members from each and with the chairman from Tulane.

The Tulane hospital had been built to accommodate the private patients of the faculty about fifteen years before the sale. It was solvent when sold, but the university was worried that medical finances would not remain as agreeable and that the support the hospital provided to the university would decrease or disappear. "The negotiating was conducted quietly and concluded rather quickly," remembers Dr. John LaRosa, then chancellor of the Tulane medical center. "HCA lived up to everything they had agreed to do. They managed the hospital very well—wouldn't let problems fester as universities are prone to do—and the medical center's financial contributions to Tulane changed very little."[11]

"We're pleased that we sold to HCA," says Dr. Paul Whelton, who succeeded LaRosa at Tulane in 1999. HCA's purchase helped to remove the deficit the university had been accumulating from its medical center, contributed funds needed to improve the hospital, and helped to restore it after Hurricane Katrina had flooded the hospital in 2005.[10]

However, Whelton believes "HCA would probably pass on buying us today. We're a bit of a nuisance to them."[10] As is the case for Universal at GW's university hospital, Tulane's teaching hospital produces lower margins for HCA than do the company's community hospitals. Whelton fears that the company's investments in the hospital may decrease as the HCA executives take the company private and incur the usual debt for such transactions.[10,12]

University of Oklahoma

In the mid-1990s, the state of Oklahoma decided to offer its university and children's hospitals to outside entities for a long-term lease-management arrangement rather than continue paying their deficits. Operating under state auspices, the hospitals had to comply with civil services regulations unsuitable for hospitals and deal with the patronage system characteristic of the state government.

HCA was one of four enterprises that bid for the hospitals. In 1998, after two years of negotiations, the two university hospitals and the adjacent private Presbyterian Hospital, already owned by HCA, were merged through a joint operating agreement with the University Hospitals Authority and

Trust, HCA, and the University of Oklahoma. HCA would manage the three hospitals, now unified governmentally as the University of Oklahoma Medical Center. Gradually the losses were reversed and surpluses developed, the first $9 million of which would be retained in the trust and any residual above this amount divided between HCA and the trust. The state continued to support the care of indigent patients.

"Things worked pretty well until 2003," said Dr. Dewayne Andrews, dean of the college of medicine and vice president of health affairs since 2002. "Then tensions became severe as the economy dropped and the cost of care rose. HCA was 'off-budget' and hunkered down as working relationships between the medical school and the hospital system deteriorated."[13]

Andrews describes how HCA, like other for-profit hospital-owning corporations, operates financially on a short-term basis, whereas academic medical centers work on longer, one- to three-year horizons. "HCA focuses on quarterly, even thirty-day budgets," says Andrews. "If the results don't meet predictions, they enter a reactive pattern that sometimes seems almost like a panic mode. They demand margins that academic medical centers can't deliver—HCA at times wants 16 to 17 percent, for example." Also, the school could not accept the company's plan that faculty members invest in surgi-centers the company wanted to develop off campus.[13]

The union with HCA "served its purposes in 1998, and we've become much stronger," but, Andrews adds, "HCA doesn't really support clinical research, and decision making about clinical operations and educational programs has become more and more problematic. So we've got significant issues these days."[13] As at Tulane, the medical school leadership is worried about the effect on the medical center of privatizing the corporation.

The University Hospitals Trust and the school are exploring their options with respect to HCA's interest in the medical center and would consider assigning the hospitals to a new 501(c)(3) corporation.[13] "For-profits may be good for the short term, but not necessarily for the long term," Andrews has concluded.[13]

Saint Louis University

On February 24, 1998, Saint Louis University (SLU) sold its university hospital for $300 million in cash[14] to Tenet Healthcare,[15] which agreed to invest $30 million annually for five years in capital improvements for the hospital.[14]

As at the University of Southern California, governance rests with Tenet, which wholly owns the hospital through a subsidiary. Unlike at George Washington, Creighton, Oklahoma, and Tulane, the university does not own part of the subsidiary or participate directly in its governance.[16] There is a hospital board consisting of five representatives from the university and five from the community chosen by Tenet.[17] Hospital CEO Crystal Haynes describes the board as serving "in an advisory capacity responsible for quality of care, compliance, MD credentialing. It's not the traditional board you would find at a not-for-profit. It has no responsibility for budget, executive salaries, capital, fundraising, etc."[16]

Although the hospital had revenue of $194 million and had generated a surplus of $30 million on operations in the year before the sale,[18] "we hadn't developed a hospital system as some of the others in town had done," explains Father Lawrence Biondi, S.J., the university president.[19] He and the trustees worried about the future financial viability of the hospital and its school of medicine.[20]

When the university owned the hospital, its employees received academic-style benefits unsuitable to sustaining a competitive position in the market, where expenses were growing and revenue shrinking.[21] As for the medical school, Biondi was quoted by the *St. Louis Post-Dispatch* as saying that "Saint Louis University would have been forced to close its medical school within 10 years had it accepted a $200 million bid [$100 million less than what Tenet paid] for SLU hospital from the area's two Catholic hospital systems."[14]* The president looked on the sale as a means of increasing the university's endowment with the proceeds directed to the school.[20] Until Tenet would make enough money from the hospital to direct some funds to the medical school, the income from the endowment would "offset what the hospital's profits had been adding to the university," says James Kimmey.[21]†

Completing the sale required overcoming opposition from the archbishop of St. Louis[22] and the Vatican,[23] which viewed with growing concern the intrusion of for-profit companies into health care.[15] Although founded

---

* "Tenet paid more than the hospital was worth at the time," believes James Kimmey, vice president for health sciences and chief executive officer of the health sciences center from 1993 to 1998, who was in charge of the sale on behalf of the university. "They paid to buy the prestige of owning a university hospital in St. Louis,"[21] as MedStar had done at Georgetown.

† Kimmey is now president and chief executive officer of the Missouri Foundation for Health, which he describes as the "state's largest health foundation with assets of more than $1 billion."[21]

as a Jesuit institution and with a Jesuit priest as its president, the board and Father Biondi took the point of view that the university was bound by civil law, not canon law, since its lay trustees held title to the university's assets.[14] Though the St. Louis University Hospital—the name did not change— would no longer be a Catholic institution, Tenet agreed to adhere to Catholic principles and practices, including barring abortions and sterilizations.[15] Biondi joined the Tenet board.[24]

Although consumer groups demanded that SLU spend a significant portion of the proceeds from the sale on direct health care for the poor, the university announced that the money would be used solely to strengthen the university's programs in the health professions.[17]

Unlike at Georgetown and George Washington, the practice plan for full-time physicians would remain and has remained a part of the Saint Louis University School of Medicine,[25] so the doctors' benefits have not changed as they did at Georgetown. However, that was not the case for the hospital employees, who became Tenet employees. According to the *Post Dispatch*, "St. Louis University hospital employees will lose benefits worth from a few thousand to tens of thousands of dollars."[26]

The hospital pays the school for the care that members of the clinical faculty give to charity patients and supports the costs of some unfunded research, according to Crystal Haynes, the CEO, who applauds the medical school's having its own practice plan. The provisions of the sale required that when the hospital's surpluses exceeded a certain amount, Tenet would share the remainder with the school.[21] "Right now, "she says, "we're having the most comfortable time in our relationship. We keep an eye on each other, and it works."[27]

Not everyone agrees. Dr. Adrian Di Bisceglie, the acting chairman of the department of internal medicine in 2006, observed that Tenet has become "a less agreeable partner during the past three to four years."[20] Fighting lawsuits and paying awards in recent years appears to have caused Tenet to pursue a more cautious financial policy. Obtaining Tenet support for projects the school believes wise has become more difficult,[20] and, consequently, some members of the faculty complain that the company is no longer sending enough money to the school.[21]*

*In 2006, Tenet also owned one community hospital in St. Louis in addition to the university hospital. Five hospitals in the city had been Tenet hospitals previously.[24] Another for-profit company owns two hospitals in St. Louis.[16]

Drexel University

In October 1998, Tenet Healthcare bought eight hospitals in Philadelphia, including three primary teaching hospitals: Hahnemann University Hospital, Medical College of Pennsylvania (MCP) Hospital, and St. Christopher's Hospital for Children.[28] The seller was the Allegheny Education and Research Foundation (AHERF), a not-for-profit integrated delivery system, which originated in the Allegheny Hospital in Pittsburgh and had expanded rapidly during the 1990s, purchasing hospitals and physician practices in the Philadelphia area and elsewhere.

AHERF also bought Hahnemann University, with its schools of medicine, nursing, public health, and health professions, and the Medical College of Pennsylvania and assigned them to a new subsidiary, the Allegheny University of the Health Sciences. The company then consolidated the two medical schools into a single entity called the MCP Hahnemann School of Medicine.

Extravagantly overspending its resources, AHERF filed for bankruptcy in July 1998, jeopardizing the future of the united medical school.* The medical school was taken over by Drexel University† and is now known as the Drexel University College of Medicine.[31,32] Tenet retained ownership of the MCP-Hahnemann real estate, and Drexel pays rent for use of the medical school facilities there.[33] As part of the deal, the bankruptcy creditor's committee gave Drexel $50 million for its endowment.[34]

As Tenet's financial problems mounted, the company decided to close the MCP Hospital, which was chronically losing money[35]—as much as $5 million per month.[24] Public opposition to the closure was strong, but the hospital was eventually shut down and the property sold to a local non-for-profit partnership that agreed to keep at least a hundred thousand square feet available for medical services.[36] By 2006, Tenet had sold three of the eight hospitals it once owned in Philadelphia and was trying to sell three more.[34] The company retained ownership of only Hahnemann and St. Christopher's hospitals, both of which are affiliated with the Drexel medical college[31] and both of which are profitable.[32]

---

*See the study of the Allegheny debacle by Professor Robert Burns and colleagues from the University of Pennsylvania's Wharton School.[29]

†Called the Drexel Institute of Art, Science, and Industry when it was founded in 1891 by the financier Anthony J. Drexel. It achieved university status in 1969. Drexel's president, Constantine Papadakis, likes to describe Drexel as "Philadelphia's technological university."[30]

Although Tenet's recent troubles have meant less money for capital investment in the two teaching hospitals that Tenet owns in Philadelphia, "our partnership's working very well," said Papadakis. "Of course, the relationship between a not-for-profit university and its doctors with a for-profit hospital company can be a difficult mix, a push-pull situation," he adds.[32]*

*The full-time faculty's practice plan at Drexel is associated with the medical college, not with Tenet.

Reducing Deficits and Increasing Surpluses in Private Medical Schools That Do Not Own Their Primary Teaching Hospitals

As we have seen, it was severe financial losses and accumulated deficits in their medical centers that forced George Washington and Georgetown universities to sell their hospitals and practice plans. Repairing losses in hospitals is beyond my competence, but converting red ink into black ink at medical schools and their departments is a subject with which I have had some experience. To learn more, I interviewed thirty knowledgeable people—deans, chief financial officers of medical schools and hospitals, practice plan directors, associate deans concerned with finance and organization—at some of our leading academic medical centers and acquaintances in business. I have quoted some of them directly.[1-30]

I have limited the study to private medical schools that own their practice plans but do not own their primary teaching hospitals. These schools can suffer the greatest financial challenges because they cannot rely on regular governmental funding or assured support from their teaching hospitals.

General Concepts

I was repeatedly advised that whatever one does to reduce a deficit or increase a surplus, the faculty and its leadership must participate in the process. They must become convinced that, despite the pain that the process may produce, achieving a balanced budget or larger surplus will benefit them as well as the school. As one of my sources said, "Everything flows from individual faculty members."

Some schools have histories of annual deficits that the faculty and administration and even the university have come to accept as inevitable. This attitude must change because deficits are ultimately destructive to the missions of a school. "The reality of deficits in for-profit and not-for-profits today is that they cannot be sustained, even in the intermediate term," an investment executive wrote me.

Practice Plan Problems

The practice plan usually offers the greatest opportunity for reducing deficits and increasing surpluses in schools that do not own hospitals. Major reasons that practice plans financially underperform are:

- Collection of the income generated by the doctors is poorly managed.
- Expenses to operate the plan are excessive.
- Reporting of data to the school is incomplete or has been manipulated.
- The payer mix is disadvantageous.
- The managed care contracts pay the doctors poorly.
- Compensation of the clinical faculty members does not correlate with their activities.

Practice Plan Solutions

Improve billing and collection. This work can be performed in a centralized or decentralized system, or as a combination of the two.

In a centralized system, all functions are conducted by the central office of the practice plan. This includes operating the computer system for billing and collection, the "front end" work of capturing the data from the patient encounters, and the "back end" work of resolving delinquent bills and other post-billing issues. In several of the schools I studied, the practice plan office also conducts managed care contracting.

Supporters of the centralized approach, which include most people interviewed, say that billing, collecting, and contracting are no longer suitable work for employees not specifically trained to do this work. Employees without such skills and experience may be the only people that units such as small departments can retain for this work. The high volume of activity of a centralized system enables the school to hire better-qualified people to lead and execute the work and save money on a per unit basis. A centralized system facilitates reporting of accurate, comprehensive financial data affecting the clinical operation.

In a decentralized structure, the practice plan handles the computer system that bills and collects the money and may contract for managed care business. The departments capture and code the services and manage the post-billing issues. Supporters of decentralized billing say that this approach lets departments do what they know best since billing practices vary between departments with high-volume/low-return ratios like medicine and pediatrics and low-volume/high-return ratios like surgery. In one school I contacted that favors a centralized system, some departments whose financial functions are particularly well managed have remained decentralized.

Converting from decentralized to centralized systems predictably arouses territorial objections from chairmen and their administrators. To reduce this tension, the school should do it gradually. Bring each department aboard one by one, starting with small departments, particularly ones that are in deficit. This gives the practice plan time to refine the system before large amounts of money are put at risk. The conversion must be conducted carefully. A poorly managed conversion can bring disastrous financial results, as was demonstrated when one of our leading medical schools tried to do this all at once ten years ago.[31]

No one interviewed favored outsourcing this function to for-profit companies.

Managed care. The plan and not individual departments should negotiate for managed care contracts. "The more you're consolidated, the more clout you have." Some advise negotiating with the hospital for managed care business to take advantage of size and for convenience of the insurers. Others caution that the practice plan may emerge second best when so doing. Contracts that pay poorly should be rejected.

Raise fees for medical services. One source said that, in his school, some departments had not raised their fees "for years."

Raise the dean's tax on clinical income. An unpopular but, in the case of a school-wide deficit, a decision to be considered.

Outpatient offices. Practice plans can shed up to 10 percent of costs by seeing patients in hospital-based facilities rather than in units run by practice plans.

Compensation of clinical faculty. (See mission-based compensation below.)

Central Administrative Structure

Create a fiscal affairs advisory committee that reviews departmental financial data to assure progress of each unit toward meeting its financial, administrative, and academic goals. Since chairmen and directors often see centralization of financial and administrative functions in the dean's office as interfering with their responsibilities, it is vital that they be involved in the process of developing and then maintaining a debt-free, surplus-producing medical school through a mechanism like a fiscal affairs advisory committee.

The group should pay particular attention to departments in deficit. All financial data should be available for review, including how much the dean supports each department and departmental, but not individual, compensation.

The committee should help the school decide in what order the deficit-reducing, surplus-enhancing repairs should be undertaken. Only one or just a few projects should be operating simultaneously. Less controversial projects should be undertaken first.

If the group functions well, chairmen will learn from each other about their successes as well as their mistakes and collaborate in solving financial issues. No chairman will be able to sustain an undercover deal or retain an untouchable "sacred cow" if all data are available and subject to the force of peer review.

As for size, one school uses a committee of six to eight chairmen. At another, the committee includes all the chairmen. At each school, the groups meets monthly.

Accounting. All funds accounting systems should be instituted and refined so that the school and the departments receive all the data they need. The information should be presented in a similar form to all units. Establishing an all funds system is not complicated, I was told. "All funds is not rocket science, just good, comprehensive accounting."*

The school, including the practice plan, should try to use accrual accounting even though cash-based accounting is superficially easier to understand. Accrual accounting "gets rid of artificial timing complications," as one of the CPAs I spoke with said. If the hospital also uses accrual accounting, as most hospitals do, financial clarity will improve when the medical school uses the same system.

Reports should include income and expense statements, balance sheets, and statements of cash flow.

Reducing Expenses

Mission-based compensation. Faculty salaries are usually the largest cost in those medical schools that are based on a full-time system and do not own

---

*See W. R. Elger, who describes how the University of Michigan School of Medicine approached this project.[32]

hospitals. Consequently, they offer significant opportunities for saving. Managing this process, however, can be difficult, time consuming, and, in some cases, painful.

Faculty should be paid according to their productivity in clinical practice, education, research, and administration. The system should be applied to all faculty members whether or not their department or division is in deficit. "Faculty must cover their salaries for a school to turn around," I was advised. "If they don't, you're lost."

The process should start at the department level with annual reviews of each faculty member and administrator. After receiving the chairmen's recommendations, the dean should also review the financial condition of each faculty member: net income (after all reductions) versus gross compensation (salary plus the costs of all benefits). Profit and loss statements generated for each faculty member will facilitate the process.

Develop a workable plan to establish base salaries, supplements, and bonuses that all members of the faculty can understand and live with. As one source said, "Salary deals are often set in backrooms. Not wise." Successful faculty members do not like to learn that the salaries of their less productive colleagues rise the same amount as theirs.

The custom of maintaining salaries from year to year—as if they were guaranteed not to fall—will tend to perpetuate a deficit.

Standardize, as much as possible, the financial benefits that faculty members and nonprofessional employees receive. The dean should approve all changes in benefit programs.

Consolidate administrative and support staff. At one leading medical school, the chief financial officer has amalgamated administration in pediatrics, family medicine, and clinical genetics; surgery and orthopedics; anesthesiology and emergency medicine; biomathematics and neurobiology (the only merger in basic science so far). She expects to consolidate the administration of more departments and divisions in the near future. One secretary suffices for three faculty members in the basic science departments at another school. At Georgetown, the administration of all the basic science departments has been consolidated in one office.*

Try to use benchmarks for evaluating the effectiveness of administrative activity as hospitals do.

*See chapter 8.

Consider locating administrative offices where costs are lower than in laboratory or hospital space.

Close or reduce the size of deficit-producing units. The strategy of closing financially draining medical units is anathema to medical schools, which have long believed that they must provide medical services in all the specialties. Yet this may be necessary to help reverse a school's deficit. The school's leadership should ask themselves, "Why are we supporting this unit? Are we involved in an activity that loses money but doesn't help our mission?" Several of my non-M.D. sources wished that their deans would close departments that were perpetually in deficit—vertical cutting—rather than reducing costs across the school—horizontal cutting. If one decides not to close such programs, consider reducing their size.

Familiar examples of this problem, which can contribute significantly to deficits in medical schools, are the practices of non-procedure-performing, outpatient clinicians, such as family practice, general internal medicine, endocrinology, rheumatology, diabetes, general pediatrics, several of the nonprocedural pediatrics divisions, and certain divisions in obstetrics, neurology, and psychiatry. Without subsidies, most of these units cannot avoid losing money.

Some suggest that schools should separate these clinicians from the full-time system and let them run their own practices, thereby transferring the financial risks from the school to them. The principal monetary disadvantage of this change is the potential loss of the income generated from the office procedures they order and the downstream revenue their practices generate. The risk of losing this potential income might persuade the hospital's leaders to better subsidize such money-losing operations.

Receivership. Put departments that are losing money into what amounts to receivership and severely limit their ability to spend until the deficit is eliminated. The fiscal affairs advisory committee should review frequently the financial status of departments in this condition.

Unbudgeted spending. Faculty and administrators should receive permission from the fiscal affairs advisory committee or the dean before spending sizeable unbudgeted funds.

Malpractice insurance. Study whether the practice plan can obtain more cost-efficient malpractice insurance. Consider linking the doctors' insurance to that of the hospital. Sometimes this association can be beneficial.

Cost of benefits. Review insurance and workmen's compensation policies.

Can similar protection be obtained for lower premiums from other companies? Provide a financial incentive for employees whose spouses have superior health care policies to relinquish their own policies.

Space. Reduce the fixed cost of maintaining offices and laboratories by closing those that are empty, consolidating those that are not maximally utilized, and leasing unused labs to other entities.

Consider leasing space rather than constructing new laboratory buildings. "A five-year lease can be easier to deal with than thirty years of debt service."

Make more efficient use of space not owned by the medical school for doctors' offices. Negotiate to reduce the rent.

Consider working with a developer to generate new income-producing space on the medical school campus.

Overhead. Raising the rate of recovery of indirect costs can be a good source of additional income in medical schools with strong science. The current amount collected may not cover all the costs for the research being funded.

Telephone. Can the cost that the local and long-distance providers charge be reduced by changing companies? Encourage faculty and staff to be more economical, particularly in the use of cell phones and similar devices. Consider installing a system that monitors the cost of long-distance calls.

Purchasing. Reduce the cost of supplies purchased by the school for the departments and divisions by buying in bulk and convincing vendors to reduce their prices. The school may want to employ a purchasing agent to make such a program maximally effective. When cash is needed, delay paying suppliers.

Payments to the university. Renegotiate the amount the university requires the school to pay if it is more than the true costs of the services the university provides.

Debt to the university. If the university is holding the medical school responsible for accumulated deficits (in effect, a loan), try to convince the university to forgive all or part of the loan, using as an argument the school's efforts to reduce its present deficit. Of the amount that remains, try to restructure the loan by repaying it over a longer term. If interest is being charged, try to have it reduced.

Increase Income by Convincing the Principal Teaching Hospital to Better Support the School

Few private medical schools can sustain themselves on professional income, grants, overhead, tuition, and philanthropy alone. Consequently, for the school to thrive, the hospital, "the real economic engine in medical centers," must transfer—not "subsidize," insisted one of my sources—to the school more money than what it pays for the professional and administrative services it purchases. The hospital must understand and accept that part of the transfer may support education and basic research in addition to clinical programs. Without hospital money, few private schools can afford to recruit and retain superior faculty, make renovations, or build new facilities.*

Unfortunately, as one of my sources said, "the leaders of most teaching hospitals give the school and its faculty less credit than they deserve for making the hospital work." All too few hospital executives acknowledge that "nothing happens in a hospital until a doctor does something—admits a patient, performs an operation, orders a test, or prescribes a drug," a hospital CFO told me. Consequently, he added, "docs have enormous influence on the success of hospitals."

So why should hospitals provide this support? Many primary teaching hospitals without their associated medical schools would just look like large community hospitals, often because of their long histories and because they are located in down-market sections of their cities, which many of the city's better-insured citizens do not frequent. Schools should take advantage of this reality by continuously emphasizing how much the medical school and its faculty enhance the success and reputation of the hospital. This requires repetitive reinforcement at the highest levels between the CEO of the hospital, the dean, and the president of the university, and among trustees of both institutions.

Transparency. Several sources emphasized the importance of building the school-hospital relationship on the basis of total transparency so that the

---

*Here are two examples at leading academic medical centers in which the hospital assists the medical school. In St. Louis, Barnes-Jewish and St. Louis Children's hospitals give the medical school at Washington University 45 percent of their combined operating margins.[30] In Baltimore, the Johns Hopkins and Bayview hospitals—both are parts of the Johns Hopkins Health System—send $75 million annually to the Johns Hopkins University School of Medicine for services given, each of which, explains the dean Dr. Edward Miller, is "well documented."[33] For example, the hospital pays half of the salaries of the [clinical] department chairmen.

hospital knows how the school is doing and the school understands where the hospital is having troubles as well as enjoying successes. A teaching hospital CFO complained bitterly about not knowing why one of the clinical departments was losing money because the school refused to share the information. "Made us think twice about supporting some of their projects," he said to me. When transparency replaces secrecy, trust grows, leading to greater success for both parties and greater likelihood that the hospital will rely on the school to spend its funds wisely and economically.

The chairmen and their faculty should know just how much money the hospital is providing. This knowledge will reduce the faculty's sense that the hospital is not helping enough and, by making the data public, pressure the hospital to help more, particularly if its support is less than generous.

Comparisons. Deans may be able to further convince hospital executives to increase their financial help by showing them data from those institutions where the hospital-to-school transfers are greater and by reminding them that the stronger the school becomes, the greater the hospital can become.

Schools in deficit are a risk to teaching hospitals. To counter the tendency of hospital executives to question the competence of the leadership of a such a school, the dean must assure the hospital that he is working effectively to reverse the losses. This will reduce their concern that the funds the hospital invests in school-sponsored programs are "just flowing into that black hole over at the school," as one of my sources put it. Hospital executives are understandably wary of investing in schools that are not operating efficiently. As a hospital CFO told me, "The hospital will suffer economically whenever the school and its docs aren't doing well economically and academically."

Administration. Evaluate whether the hospital is adequately supporting the school for the time members of the faculty spend administering hospital laboratories and services, teaching the residents, directing the nurses, and participating in the work of hospital committees.

Business plans. Every new proposal for hospital support should be developed from a professional, persuasive business plan that will convince the hospital that the new program will benefit the hospital as well as the school. Every proposal must give the hospital value for money. Success more likely follows if the proposal is presented with the words, "let's do this together."

Proposals should be negotiated between chairmen and the hospital director. A division head or laboratory director on the school side and junior executives from the hospital may help develop programs, but the final discussions should be conducted in the presence of the senior leaders.

A representative from the dean's office should participate in these meetings, showing that the school is intimately involved in the process and that the service chief is not operating on his own. The hospital may respond more favorably to proposals when it realizes that the school is energetically and effectively reducing the deficit if it has one.

Hospital's capital program. Joint planning is especially necessary in the assignment of the capital program. As a rule, I was told, hospitals allot about 60 percent of capital funds to the strategic objectives and 40 percent to internal improvements, such as repairing or replacing obsolete facilities and improving information technology.

Increasing Income by Other Methods

Increase the overhead recovery rate. With energy and construction costs rising rapidly, a cogent argument can be made for trying to convince the NIH and other agencies to do this.

Increase the endowment. Create a development office if the school does not already have one. In many universities, these offices are satellites of the central development department. This can work well so long as the personnel in the school are highly competent.

Biotechnology transfer. Particularly in schools with strong science programs, create a professional office that assists investigators in bringing their discoveries to market.

Incentives

Provide incentives to encourage faculty members to demonstrate their inherent skills, ingenuity, and drive to succeed.

Emphasize individual incentives. Group incentives can also help.

Salary from grants. Let the investigators retain a portion of what they generate in salary support. To retain this money, investigators, particularly in the basic sciences but also in the clinical departments, should develop more of their salaries from grants. Set individual targets for salary support for faculty based on their experience and seniority and average targets for departments.

Let departments keep surpluses, or a portion of them, as an incentive to increase income and reduce expenses.

Overheads. Here's a provocative approach one of the sources advised. Send the overhead funds, minus a portion retained in the dean's office, to the departments in proportion to the grants their faculty develop. Charge the departments for the expenses the overhead is intended to cover on a square-foot basis. Let the department keep any surplus. The chairmen and colleagues will come to understand that space is a resource that costs money and will be challenged to maximize the use of this money by using his space more economically. If this idea appeals, start by testing it in one basic science department.

Some Principles

Do not invade the capital of the endowment to pay for operating losses.

Growth by itself will not reduce a deficit. Despite adding people and programs, the problems that are causing the deficit will remain. Every young clinician needs money to get started, and new investigators must be sustained until the grants come in.

With federal limits on support for investigators' salaries, it will cost the school money to add all but a few very well-funded investigators, let alone an investigator without adequate support. The research enterprise can require a subsidy of as much as 30 percent, which means that, as research activity grows, "the school becomes increasingly leveraged." Faculty members should not be supported indefinitely to perform unfunded research. "Research is a negative cash-flow business," as several sources reminded me in so many words.

Growth alone can help, however, when expanding programs use fixed costs more efficiently.

Using consultants. All my sources agree that consultants should be employed sparingly and that implementation of whatever advice they give should be carried out internally whenever possible. Hiring consultants may be necessary, however, when the staff of the school does not have the experience needed to accomplish a task. One source advised letting the consultant be the "bad guy" if the advice, though wise, will be unpalatable to the staff or faculty.

To reduce the expense, consultants should be retained:

- On the basis of their response to a request for proposal (RFP).
- On a contingency basis so that part of their fee depends on the success of the mission.
- By carefully defining the scope of the engagement.
- By keeping the consulting team on target by meeting weekly with the principal of the consulting firm assigned to the job.
- By limiting expenses to a fraction of the total contract and/or specifying what hotel they use, how much they spend for food and transportation, etc.

Caution

Some members of the faculty will oppose instituting the changes discussed in this document and, when the changes strike home, may even try to have the dean dismissed. Consequently, it is essential that the university leadership approve the strategy and support the dean in the changes he will make.

Interviewees

Past and present titles at George Washington, Georgetown, and MedStar are listed first. Titles without dates are those held when the interviews were conducted. Locations are in Washington, D.C., unless otherwise indicated.

CEO = chief executive officer; CFO = chief financial officer; CNMC = Children's National Medical Center; COO = chief operating officer; EVP = executive vice president; GU = Georgetown University; GUH = Georgetown University Hospital; GUMC = Georgetown University Medical Center; GWUSPH = George Washington University School of Public Health and Health Services; GWU = George Washington University; GWUH = George Washington University Hospital; GWUMC = George Washington University Medical Center; GWUSM = George Washington University School of Medicine; Lombardi = Lombardi Comprehensive Cancer Center; MFA = George Washington University Medical Faculty Associates; MedStar = MedStar Health; SUNY = State University of New York; UMSM = University of Maryland School of Medicine; VP = vice president; WHC = Washington Hospital Center

NAME	POSITION
Adashi, Eli Y., M.D.	Dean of Medicine and Biological Sciences, Brown University, Providence, RI
Adkins, Mark S., M.D.	Clinical Chief of Cardiac Surgery, GWUH (1999–2004); Professor of Clinical Cardiothoracic Surgery, Weill Medical College of Cornell University; Chairman, Department of Cardiothoracic Surgery, New York Hospital, Queens, New York, NY
Adkison, Claudia R., J.D., Ph.D.	Executive Associate Dean, Administration and Faculty Affairs, Emory University School of Medicine, Atlanta, GA

Akman, Jeffrey S., M.D.	Chairman, Department of Psychiatry, GWUSM
Alcorn, Karen M.	VP, Public Affairs, GUH
Alpern, Robert J., M.D.	Dean, Yale University School of Medicine, New Haven, CT
Amsterdam, Philip S.	Trustee, GWU
Anderson, Minor W.	Various administrative positions, GUMC (1993–2000); Associate VP for Medical Affairs and Managing Director, University of Miami Medical Group, Miami, FL
Andrews, M. Dewayne, M.D.	Executive Dean and VP for Health Affairs, University of Oklahoma College of Medicine, Oklahoma City, OK
Antman, Karen H., M.D.	Provost, Boston University Medical Campus and Dean, Boston University School of Medicine, Boston, MA
Applegate, William B., M.D.	Senior VP, Wake Forest University Health Sciences and Dean, Wake Forest University School of Medicine, Winston-Salem, NC
Areen, Judith C., J.D.	Paul Regis Dean Professor of Law and Dean Emerita, GU Law Center
Aronovitch, Stanley, D.Sc.	CEO, GWU Health Plan (1998–2001); President and CEO, Mercy Care Plan, Phoenix, AZ
Badger, Stephen L.	CEO, Medical Faculty Associates
Bailey, David N., M.D.	Interim Vice Chancellor for Health Sciences and Interim Dean, University of California, San Diego School of Medicine, San Diego, CA
Balke, C. William, M.D.	Senior Associate Dean for Research, University of Kentucky College of Medicine, Lexington, KY
Barch, Michael M.	CEO, GWUH (1978–90); Chairman, Global Pharmaceutical Sourcing, Bethesda, MD

Barchi, Robert L., M.D., Ph.D.	President, Thomas Jefferson University, Philadelphia, PA
Barish, Robert A., M.D.	Associate Dean for Clinical Affairs, UMSOM
Barnes, Anne C.	Associate Dean for Finance, University of Oklahoma College of Medicine, Oklahoma City, OK
Barnhill, Raymond L., M.D.	Chairman, Department of Dermatology, GWUSM (2002–4); Clinical Professor of Dermatology and Pathology, University of Miami Miller School of Medicine; Senior Dermatopathologist, Global Pathology Laboratory Services, Inc., Miami Lakes, FL
Bass, Gerald H.	Associate VP for Health Economics, GWUMC
Batshaw, Mark L., M.D.	Professor and Chairman, Department of Pediatrics, GWUSM; Chief Academic Officer and Director, Children's Research Institute, CNMC
Becker, Richard B., M.D.	CEO, GWUH
Benson, Nicholas, M.D.	Vice Dean and Senior Associate Dean for Operations, Brody School of Medicine of East Carolina University, Greenville, NC
Berg, Patricia E., Ph.D.	Associate Professor of Biochemistry and Molecular Biology, GWUSM
Bergin, Adrian	Executive Administrator, Departments of Obstetrics and Gynecology and Pediatrics, GUMC (1994–98); Senior Administrator, Department of Obstetrics and Gynecology, University of Maryland School of Medicine, Baltimore, MD
Berk, Steven L., M.D.	Dean, Texas Tech Health Science Center School of Medicine, Lubbock, TX
Berrigan, Michael J., M.D.	Chairman, Department of Anesthesiology and Critical Care Medicine, GWUSM

Bing, Debbie — Principal, Center for Applied Research (CFAR), Philadelphia, PA

Biondi, Lawrence H., S.J., Ph.D. — President, St. Louis University, St. Louis, MO

Birnbaum, Philip S., M.D. — Dean Emeritus of the Medical Center for Administrative Affairs, GWUMC

Bjorkman, David J., M.D. — Dean, University of Utah School of Medicine, Salt Lake City, UT

Black, Michael E. — Associate Vice Chancellor for Administration and Finance, Washington University in St. Louis School of Medicine, St. Louis, MO

Blake, David A. — Consultant

Bloem, Kenneth D. — CEO, GUMC (1996–99)

Bondurant, Stuart, M.D. — Interim EVP for Health Sciences and Executive Dean, GUMC; Professor of Medicine and Dean Emeritus, University of North Carolina School of Medicine (1997–2004)

Bowles, L. Thompson, M.D. — EVP, GWUMC (1987–92)

Boyden, Jaclyne W. — Deputy Dean for Finance and Administration, Yale University School of Medicine, New Haven, CT

Brady, Luther W., Jr., M.D. — Emeritus Trustee, GWU; Distinguished University Professor, Drexel University College of Medicine, Philadelphia, PA

Brand, Joseph L., J.D. — Emeritus Trustee, GHU; Partner, Patton Boggs

Breault, Patrick W. — Administrator, Department of Medicine, UMSOM

Brown, Ronald A. — Administrator, Department of Pediatrics, GUMC (1998–2004); Senior Administrator, Department of Surgery, University of Maryland School of Medicine

Buja, L. Maximilian, M.D. — EVP for Academic Affairs, University of Texas Health Science Center at Houston, Houston, TX

Cain, Michael E., M.D.	Dean, School of Medicine and Biomedical Sciences, University of Buffalo, SUNY, Buffalo, NY
Calderone, Richard A., Ph.D.	Chairman, Department of Microbiology and Immunology, GUMC
Campbell, Karen, Ph.D.	Vice Chair, Department of Medicine and Administrator, Department of Neurology, GUMC (1992–2001); Executive Director, American Society of Nephrology
Caputy, Anthony J., M.D.	Chairman, Department of Neurosurgery, GWUSM
Carbonell, Nelson A., Jr.	Trustee, GWU; President and Chairman, Snowbird Capital, Reston, VA
Carpenter, Bernard A.	Associate Dean for Practice Affairs, University of Maryland School of Medicine, Baltimore, MD
Carr, Oliver T., Jr.	Chairman of the Board of Trustees Emeritus, GWU; Chairman, The Oliver Carr Company
Cassem, Edwin H., S.J., M.D.	Director, GU (1990–2004); Professor of Psychiatry, Harvard Medical School and Psychiatrist, Massachusetts General Hospital, Boston, MA
Cavender, Laura S.	Executive Director, Communications, GUMC
Cerqueira, Manuel D., M.D.	Chairman, Molecular and Functional Imaging, Cleveland Clinic Foundation, Cleveland, OH; Director, Nuclear Cardiology, Exercise Stress Testing Laboratory and Cardiac Rehabilitation, GUMC (1994–2004); Chief of Cardiology, GUMC (2003–4)
Cesario, Thomas C., M.D.	Dean, University of California, Irvine College of Medicine, Irvine, CA
Chapman, Thomas W., Ed.D.	CEO, GWUH (1994–96); President and CEO, The HSC Foundation

Chaufournier, Roger L.

Various positions, GWUH and GWUMC (1981–93); President and CEO, Center for Strategic Innovation, Bethesda, MD

Chiappinelli, Vincent A., Ph.D.

Chairman, Department of Pharmacology and Physiology, GWUSM

Chrencik, Robert A.

EVP and CFO, University of Maryland Medical System, Baltimore, Baltimore, MD

Churchill, Winston J., J.D.

Director, GU; Director, MedStar; Managing General Partner, SCP Private Equity Partners, L.P., Wayne, PA

Clauw, Daniel J., M.D.

Chief, Division of Rheumatology, Immunology, and Allergy (1997–2002) and Vice Chair, Department of Medicine, GUMC (2000–2002); Professor of Medicine, Division of Rheumatology, University of Michigan, Ann Arbor, MI

Clough, E. Craig

Associate VP for Operations and COO, GWUH (1993–97); COO, University Physicians Medical Group Practice and Kentucky Clinic Administration, Lexington, KY

Cohen, Marcia J.

Senior Associate Dean, Finance and Administration, Stanford University School of Medicine, Stanford, CA

Cohen, Sheldon S., J.D.

Chairman of the Board of Trustees Emeritus, GWU; Director, Farr, Miller & Washington

Colenda, Christopher C., M.D.

Dean, Texas A&M Health Science Center College of Medicine, College Station, TX

Corn, Milton, M.D.

Dean, GUMC (1985–89); Associate Director of Extramural Programs, National Library of Medicine, Bethesda, MD

Corso, Paul J., M.D.

Clinical Professor of Surgery, GUMC and GWUSM; Director, Section of Cardiac Surgery, WHC; Director, MedStar

Cosgrove, Delos M., M.D. CEO, Cleveland Clinic Foundation, Cleveland, OH

Cossman, Jeffrey, M.D. Chairman, Department of Pathology, GUMC (1989–97); Chief Scientific Officer, The Critical Path Institute, Rockville, MD

Cox, James L., M.D. Chief of Cardiac Surgery, Department of Surgery, GUMC (1997–2000)

Crandall, Edward D., M.D., Ph.D. Chairman, Department of Medicine, Keck School of Medicine, University of Southern California, Los Angeles, CA

Cullen, Kevin J., M.D. Interim Director, Lombardi, GUMC (2000–2002); Director, University of Maryland Greenebaum Cancer Center, Baltimore, MD

Cupples, Howard P., M.D. Professor Emeritus of Ophthalmology, GUMC; Chairman, Department of Ophthalmology, GUMC (2003–5)

Curran, Michael J. EVP and CFO, MedStar

Curzan, Myron P. Trustee, GWU; CEO, UniDev LLC, Bethesda, MD

Daroff, Robert B., M.D. Interim Chairman of Neurology, Case Western Reserve School of Medicine, Cleveland, OH

Davidson, Bruce J., M.D. Chairman, Department of Otolaryngology—Head and Neck Surgery, GUMC

Davis, F. Daniel, Ph.D. Various academic and administrative positions, GU, GUMC, GUMC (1984–2005); Executive Director, President's Council on Bioethics

Deckers, Peter J., M.D. EVP for Health Affairs and Dean, University of Connecticut School of Medicine, Farmington, CT

Deeley, John M. Executive Dean for Administration, BioMed Medical Affairs, Brown University, Providence, RI

DeGioia, John J., Ph.D. President, GU

Diamond, Louis H., M.D.　Chairman, Georgetown Department of Medicine, DC General Hospital, GUMC (1981–93); Professor of Medicine, GUMC (1987–93); Medical Director and VP, MedStar

DiBisceglie, Adrian M., M.D.　Acting Chairman, Department of Internal Medicine, Saint Louis University, St. Louis, MO

Dimolitsas, Spiros, Ph.D.　Senior VP and Chief Administrative Officer, GU

Dismuke, S. Edwards, M.D.　Dean, University of Kansas School of Medicine, Wichita, KS

Dorsey, J. Kevin, M.D., Ph.D.　Dean and Provost, Southern Illinois University School of Medicine, Springfield, IL

Drass, M. Joy, M.D.　President, GUH

Drees, Betty M., M.D　Dean, University of Missouri–Kansas City School of Medicine, Kansas City, MO

Dretchen, Kenneth L., Ph.D.　Chairman, Department of Pharmacology, GUMC

Dritschilo, Anatoly, M.D.　Interim Director, Lombardi; Interim Chairman, Department of Oncology, GUMC

Dunn, Michael J., M.D.　Dean and EVP, Medical College of Wisconsin, Milwaukee, WI

Dym, Martin O., Ph.D.　Professor of Biochemistry, Molecular, and Cellular Biology

El-Bayoumi, Jehan (Gigi), M.D.　Internal Medicine Program Director, Department of Medicine, GWUSM

Elger, William R.　Executive Director, Administration and CFO, University of Michigan Medical School, Ann Arbor, MI

Elliott, Lloyd H., Ed.D.　President, GWU (1965–88)

Elting, Jeffrey A., M.D.　Medical Director, District of Columbia Hospital Association

Enarson, Cam E., M.D.　Dean, Creighton University School of Medicine and VP for Health Affairs, Creighton University, Omaha, NE

Epstein, Stephen, M.D.   Director, Cardiovascular Research
                                Institute, MedStar

Epstein, Steven A., M.D.   Chairman, Department of Psychiatry,
                                GUMC

Evans, Stephen R. T., M.D.   Chairman, Department of Surgery,
                                GUMC

Faden, Alan I., M.D.   Professor of Neurology, Neuroscience,
                                and Pharmacology, GUMC

Faselis, Charles J., M.D.   Associate Chairman and Program
                                Director, Department of Internal
                                Medicine, Veterans Administration
                                Medical Center, Washington, DC;
                                Associate Professor of Medicine,
                                GWUSM

Federman, Daniel D., M.D.   Senior Dean for Alumni Relations and
                                Clinical Teaching, Harvard Medical
                                School, Boston, MA

Ferguson, Bruce   Associate VP and CFO, UW Medicine,
                                Seattle, WA

Filerman, Gary L., Ph.D.   Chairman, Department of Health Sys-
                                tems Administration, GU School of
                                Nursing and Health Studies

Fine, Richard N., M.D.   Dean, SUNY Stony Brook School of
                                Medicine, Stony Brook, NY

Fiser, Debra H., M.D.   Dean, University of Arkansas College
                                of Medicine, Little Rock, AR

Flynn Hollander, Sharon M.   CEO, GUH (1997–2000); EVP, COO,
                                and Lead, The Hollander Group

Fogarty, John P., M.D.   Interim Dean, University of Vermont
                                College of Medicine, Burlington, VT

Ford, Nelson M.   COO, GUMC (1992–97); Principal
                                Deputy Assistant Secretary for
                                Financial Management and Comp-
                                troller, Department of the Army

Franks, Ronald D., M.D.   VP of Health Affairs and Dean, Quillen
                                College of Medicine of East Ten-
                                nessee State University, Johnson
                                City, TN

Freedman, Michael G.   VP for Communications, GWU

Furnstahl, Lawrence J. — Chief Financial and Strategy Officer, University of Chicago Medical Center, Chicago, IL

Gabbe, Steven G., M.D. — Dean, Vanderbilt University School of Medicine, Nashville, TN

Gardner, Laurence B., M.D. — Executive Dean for Education and Policy, Leonard M. Miller School of Medicine, University of Miami, Miami, FL

Garson, Arthur T., Jr., M.D. — Dean, School of Medicine and VP, University of Virginia, Charlottesville, VA

Gersh, Bernard J., M.B., Ch.B., D.Phil. — Chief, Division of Cardiology, Department of Medicine, GUMC (1993–98); Associate Chair, Academic Affairs and Faculty Development, Mayo Clinic, Rochester, MN

Ghezzi, Keith T., M.D. — Various positions, GWUH and GWUMC (1987–96); President and CEO, Forum Health, Youngstown, OH

Gibson, J. Scott — Vice Dean, Administration and Finance, Duke University School of Medicine, Durham, NC

Gilmore, Thomas N. — VP, CFAR, Philadelphia, PA

Giordano, Joseph M., M.D. — Chairman, Department of Surgery, GWUSM

Goldberg, Richard L., M.D. — VP, Medical Affairs and Chief Medical Officer, GUH; Chairman, Department of Psychiatry, GUMC (1989–2001)

Golden, Robert N., M.D. — Dean, School of Medicine and Public Health and Vice Chancellor for Medical Affairs, University of Wisconsin, Madison, WI

Goldman, Lee, M.D. — EVP for Health and Biomedical Sciences and Dean, Faculties of Health Sciences and Medicine, Columbia University College of Physicians and Surgeons, New York, NY

Goldstein, Allan L., Ph.D.

Chairman, Department of Biochemistry and Molecular Biology, GWUSM

Greenberg, Warren, Ph.D.

Professor of Health Economics, GWUSPH

Grieco, Anthony J., M.D.

Associate Dean for Alumni Relations and Academic Events, New York University School of Medicine, New York, NY

Griffith, John F., M.D.

EVP for Health Sciences and Director, GUMC (1986–96); Executive Dean, GUMC (1989–96)

Grigsby, R. Kevin, D.S.W.

Vice Dean for Faculty and Administrative Affairs, Penn State College of Medicine, Hershey, PA

Grossi, Richard A.

CFO, Johns Hopkins Medicine

Grossman, John H., III, M.D., Ph.D.

EVP, Society for Gynecologic Investigation

Gurne, Patricia D., J.D.

Vice Chair, Board of Trustees, GWU; Managing Partner, Gurne Porter, PLLC

Guzick, David S., M.D., Ph.D.

Dean, University of Rochester School of Medicine and Dentistry, Rochester, NY

Halperin, Edward G., M.D.

Dean, University of Louisville School of Medicine, Louisville, KY

Handlir, Gregory F.

Associate Dean for Resource Management, UMSOM

Haramati, Aviad, Ph.D.

Professor of Physiology and Biophysics and Medicine, GUMC

Harris, Bradley

Chief Administrative Officer, Ohio State University School of Medicine, Columbus, OH

Hastings, Douglas, J.D.

Partner, Epstein Becker & Greene, PC

Hawkins, Sean C.

Administrator, Executive Offices, GUMC

Haynes, Crystal L.

CEO, Saint Louis University Hospital, St. Louis, MO

Headrick, Linda A., M.D.

Senior Associate Dean for Education and Faculty Development, University of Missouri—Columbia School of Medicine, Columbia, MO

Healton, Edward B., M.D.

Chairman, Department of Neurology, GUMC

Henderson, Brian E., M.D.

Dean, Keck School of Medicine of University of Southern California, Los Angeles, CA

Henrich, William L., M.D.

Dean, School of Medicine and VP for Medical Affairs, University of Texas Health Science Center at San Antonio, San Antonio, TX

Herscowitz, Herbert B., Ph.D.

Senior Associate Dean for Faculty and Academic Affairs and Professor of Microbiology, GUMC

Herzog, William, M.D.

Cardiologist, Baltimore, MD

Higginbotham, Eve J., M.D.

Dean and Senior VP for Academic Affairs, Morehouse School of Medicine, Atlanta, GA

Hindery, Michael A.

Senior Consultant, Witt/Kieffer, Palo Alto, CA; formerly Senior Associate Dean for Finance and Administration, Stanford University School of Medicine, Palo Alto, CA

Hirschhorn, Larry

Principal, Center for Applied Research (CFAR), Philadelphia, PA

Hirshfield, Anne N., Ph.D.

Associate VP for Health Research, Compliance, and Technology Transfer, GWUSM

Hochberg, Mark S., M.D.

Professor of Surgery, New York University School of Medicine, New York, NY

Hotez, Peter J., M.D., Ph.D.

Chairman, Department of Microbiology and Tropical Medicine, GWUSM

Howard, Barbara V., Ph.D.

President, MedStar Research Institute

Irani, Sands K., M.D.

Gastroenterologist, Washington, DC and Chevy Chase, MD

Jackiewicz, Thomas E.	Associate Vice Chancellor, Finance and Administration, University of California, San Diego School of Medicine, San Diego, CA
Jacobson, Robert J., M.D., B.Ch.	Interim Chairman, Department of Medicine, GUMC (1988–92); Medical Director, Palm Beach Cancer Institute Foundation, West Palm Beach, FL
Jarrell, Bruce E., M.D.	Vice Dean for Research and Academic Affairs, UMSOM
Jarrett, Thomas W., M.D.	Chairman, Department of Urology, GWUSM
Johns, Michael M. E., M.D.	EVP for Health Affairs and Director, Robert W. Woodruff Health Sciences Center and CEO, Emory Healthcare, Emory University, Atlanta, GA
Joiner, Keith A., M.D.	Dean, University of Arizona College of Medicine, Tucson, AZ
Karcher, Donald S., M.D.	Acting Chairman, Department of Pathology, GWUSM
Katz, Barrett, M.D.	Chairman, Department of Ophthalmology, GWUSM (1999–2004)
Katz, Louis H.	EVP and Treasurer, GWU
Katz, Nevin M., M.D.	Professor of Surgery, GUMC (1992–2000); Chief, Adult Cardiac Surgery, GUMC (1997–2000); Clinical Professor of Surgery, Division of Cardiothoracic Surgery, GWUSM
Katz, Paul, M.D.	Chairman, Department of Medicine, GUMC (1997–2001); COO, GUMC (1998–2000); Senior VP and Chief Medical Officer, Mount Sinai Medical Center and Miami Heart Institute, Miami Beach, FL; Professor of Medicine, University of Miami School of Medicine, Miami, FL
Katz, Richard J., M.D.	Chief, Cardiology Division, Department of Medicine, GWUSM

Katz, Ruth J., J.D.	Dean, GWUSPH
Kelly, John J., M.D.	Chairman, Department of Neurology, GWUSM
Kelly, Michael J., J.D., Ph.D.	University VP, GU (1991–98)
Kent, Kenneth M., M.D., Ph.D.	Director, Cardiac Catheterization Laboratory (1983–90) and Director, Cardiac Services (2000–2003), GUMC; Chief of Cardiology, Suburban Hospital, Bethesda, MD
Kim, Young D., M.D.	Chairman, Department of Anesthesia, GUMC
Kimmel, Jennifer, M.D.	Associate Dean for Medical Education, University of Nevada School of Medicine, Reno, NV
Kimmey, James R., M.D.	President and CEO, Missouri Foundation for Health, St. Louis, MO; VP for Health Sciences and CFO of the Health Sciences Center, St. Louis University (1993–98), St. Louis, MO
Knoll, Stanley M., M.D.	Clinical Professor of Surgery, GWUSM
Korn, David, M.D.	Senior VP, Association of American Medical Colleges
Kozera, Richard J., M.D.	Executive Associate Dean, Temple University School of Medicine, Philadelphia, PA
Krane, N. Kevin, M.D.	Vice Dean, Academic Affairs, Tulane University School of Medicine, New Orleans, LA
Kriech, Julie	Director of Finance, Health Affairs, Sanford School of Medicine, University of South Dakota, Vermillion, SD
Krugman, Richard D., M.D.	Dean, University of Colorado School of Medicine, Denver, CO
Lansberg, Lewis, M.D.	Dean and VP for Medical Affairs, Feinberg School of Medicine, Northwestern University, Chicago, IL
LaRosa, John C., M.D.	Various positions, GWUMS and GWUMC (1970–94); President, SUNY Downstate Medical Center, Brooklyn, NY

Larsen, John W., M.D.   Chairman, Department of Obstetrics
                                       and Gynecology, GWUSM

Laughlin, Larry W., M.D., Ph.D.   Dean, Uniformed Services University
                                       of the Health Sciences, F. Edward
                                       Hébert School of Medicine, Beth-
                                       esda, MD

Lazare, Aaron, M.D.   Chancellor and Dean, University of
                                       Massachusetts School of Medicine,
                                       Worcester, MA

Lazarus, Gerald S., M.D.   Trustee, GWU; Professor of Dermatol-
                                       ogy, Johns Hopkins University
                                       School of Medicine

Leapman, Stephen B., M.D.   Executive Associate Dean for Educa-
                                       tional Affairs, Indiana University
                                       School of Medicine, Indianapolis, IN

Lehman, Donald R., Ph.D.   EVP for Academic Affairs, GWU

Lemp, Michael A., M.D.   Clinical Professor of Ophthalmology,
                                       GUMC and GWUSM; Chairman,
                                       Department of Ophthalmology,
                                       GUMC (1983–92)

Leon, Martin B., M.D.   Attending Staff Cardiologist, Wash-
                                       ington Hospital Center (1990–99);
                                       Associate Director, Cardiovascular
                                       Interventional Therapy, New York–
                                       Presbyterian Hospital; Professor of
                                       Medicine, Columbia University Col-
                                       lege of Physicians and Surgeons,
                                       New York, NY

Levey, Gerald S., M.D.   Vice Chancellor for Medical Sciences
                                       and Dean, David Geffin School of
                                       Medicine at UCLA, Los Angeles, CA

Levine, Arthur S., M.D.   Senior Vice Chancellor for Health Sci-
                                       ences and Dean, University of Pitts-
                                       burgh School of Medicine, Pitts-
                                       burgh, PA

Lieberman, Steven A., M.D.   Vice Dean for Academic Affairs, Uni-
                                       versity of Texas Medical Branch,
                                       Galveston, TX

Lindor, Keith D., M.D.   Mayo Clinic College of Medicine,
                                       Rochester, MN

Lippman, Marc E.	Director, Lombardi, GUMC (1988–2001); Chairman, Department of Internal Medicine, University of Michigan Health System, Ann Arbor, MI
Lloyd, Sterling M., Jr.	Associate Dean for Administration and Planning, Howard University College of Medicine, Washington, DC
Loop, Floyd D., M.D.	CEO (1989–2004), Cleveland Clinic Foundation, Cleveland, OH
Lough, Frederick C., M.D.	Director, Cardiac Surgery, GWUH; Clinical Professor of Surgery, GWUSM
Lumpkin, Michael D., Ph.D.	Professor of Physiology and Biophysics, GUMC
Lustbader, Jay M., M.D.	Chairman, Department of Ophthalmology, GUMC
Lynch, John H., M.D.	Chairman, Department of Urology, GUMC
Manatt, Charles T., J.D.	Chairman, Board of Directors, GWU; Founder and Partner, Manatt, Phelps & Phillips
Manyak, Michael J., M.D.	Acting and Interim Chairman, Department of Urology GWUSM (1995–2005); VP for Medical Affairs, Cytogen Corporation, Princeton, NJ
Marks, Lilly	Executive Director, University Physicians, Inc. and Senior Associate Dean, Administration and Finance, University of Colorado School of Medicine, Denver, CO
Martuza, Robert L., M.D.	Chairman, Department of Neurosurgery, GUMC (1991–2000); Chief, Neurosurgery Service, Massachusetts General Hospital; Higgins Professor of Neurosurgery, Harvard Medical School
Marzano, John A.	VP, Corporate Communications, MedStar

McCaffery, Timothy A., Ph.D.	Professor of Biochemistry and Molecular Biology, GWUSM
McCartney, Cheryl F., M.D.	Executive Associate Dean for Medical Education, University of North Carolina School of Medicine, Chapel Hill, NC
McCloskey, Brian	Budget Director, Southern Illinois University School of Medicine, Springfield, IL
McConnell, John D., M.D.	EVP for Health System Affairs, University of Texas Southwestern Medical Center at Dallas, Dallas, TX
McDaniel, John P.	CEO, MedStar
McLean, Daniel P.	CEO and Managing Director, GWUH (2000–2004); Group Director, South Texas Region and CEO, South Texas Health System, Universal Heath Services
Meador, Kimford J., M.D.	Chairman, Department of Neurology, GUMC (2002–4); Melvin Greer Professor of Neurology, University of Florida, Gainesville, FL
Medina, Deborah Taylor	Director, Management Unit and Senior Executive Assistant to the Dean, University of California, San Francisco School of Medicine, San Francisco, CA
Merson, Michael R.	Various senior administrative positions at Franklin Square Hospital, Helix, BWHealth, and MedStar; currently Chairman of the Board of Directors, CareFirst, Blue Cross/ BlueShield, Owings Mills, MD
Meyer, Roger E., M.D.	VP, Medical Affairs and Executive Dean, GWUMC (1993–95); CEO, Best Practice Project Management, Inc., Bethesda, MD
Miller, Alan B.	Founder, President, and CEO, Universal Health Services, Inc., King of Prussia, PA

Miller, D. Douglas., M.D., C.M.   Dean, Medical College of Georgia School of Medicine, Augusta, GA

Miller, Edward D., M.D.   Dean, Johns Hopkins University School of Medicine; CEO, Johns Hopkins Medicine

Miller, Jeffrey C.   Senior Executive Associate Dean and COO, Feinberg School of Medicine, Northwestern University, Chicago, IL

Miller, Leslie W., M.D.   Walters Chair of Cardiovascular Medicine, GUMC; Chief, Integrated Cardiology Programs, WHC and GUH

Mitchell, Stephen Ray, M.D.   Dean for Medical Education, GUMC

Monteleone, Patricia L., M.D.   Dean, St. Louis University School of Medicine, St. Louis, MO

Montgomery Rice, Valerie, M.D.   Senior VP for Health Affairs and Dean, School of Medicine at Meharry Medical College, Nashville, TN

Morad, Martin, Ph.D.   Professor of Pharmacology and Medicine, GUMC

Morrison, Gail, M.D.   Vice Dean for Education and Director, Office of Academic Programs, University of Pennsylvania School of Medicine, Philadelphia, PA

Mount, Kenneth J.   Associate Dean for Fiscal Affairs, University of Wisconsin School of Medicine and Public Health, Madison, WI

Moxley, John H., III, M.D.   Korn/Ferry International, Los Angeles, CA

Mrazek, David A., M.D.   Professor of Psychiatry, Behavioral Sciences, and Pediatrics, GWUSM (1991–2000); Chairman, Department of Psychiatry and Psychology, Mayo Medical School, Rochester, MN

Mullan, Fitzhugh, M.D.   Murdock Head Professor of Medicine and Health Policy, GWUSPH; Clinical Professor of Pediatrics, GWUSM

Myers, Allen R., M.D.	Professor of Medicine, Temple University, Philadelphia, PA.
Nasca, Thomas J., M.D.	Dean, Jefferson Medical College, Philadelphia, PA
Nauta, Russell J., M.D.	Chief, Division of General Surgery, GUMC (1988–97); Chairman, Department of Surgery, Mount Auburn Hospital, Cambridge, MA; Professor of Surgery, Harvard Medical School, Boston, MA
Neitz, Stephen	VP, Office of the CEO, MedStar
Nelson, David B., M.D.	Chairman, Department of Pediatrics, GUMC
Neviaser, Robert J., M.D.	Chairman, Department of Orthopedics, GWUSM
Newman, Paul	Executive Director, Duke Private Diagnostic Clinic (PDC) and Duke Patient Revenue Management Organization (PRMO); VP for Ambulatory Care, Duke University Health System, Durham, NC
Nichols, David G., M.D.	Vice Dean for Education, Johns Hopkins University School of Medicine, Baltimore, MD
O'Boyle, Michael P.	CFO, MedStar (1999–2001); COO, Cleveland Clinic Foundation
O'Brien, Charles M.	Administrator and CEO, GUH (1975–92)
O'Brien, Richard L., M.D.	University Professor, Center for Health Policy and Ethics, Creighton University; Dean, Creighton University School of Medicine (1982–92), Omaha, NE
O'Leary, Dennis S., M.D.	Medical Director, GWUH (1974–86); Dean for Clinical Affairs, GWUMC and VP, GWU Health Plan (1977–86); President, Joint Commission on Accreditation of Healthcare Organizations, Oakbrook Terrace, IL
Orlowski, Janis M., M.D.	Chief Medical Officer, WHC

Ostrander, Gary K., Ph.D.	Interim Dean, John A. Burns School of Medicine, University of Hawaii, Honolulu, HI
Ott, John E., M.D.	Director, GWU Health Plan, GWUMC (1977–85, 1987–95)
Papadakis, Constantine, Ph.D.	President, Drexel University, Philadelphia, PA
Papadopoulos, Vassilios, D.Pharm., Ph.D.	Director, Biomedical Graduate Research Organization, Associate VP for Research, GUMC
Pawlson, Gregory L., M.D.	Chairman, Department of Health Care Sciences, GWUSM (1987–98)
Pearle, David L., M.D.	Director, Coronary Care Unit, GUH; Acting Chief, Division of Cardiology, GUH (1988–93)
Peartree, Louisa A.	Assistant Dean, Administration, UMSOM
Pelegrino, Edmund, M.D.	John Carroll Professor of Medicine and Medical Ethics, Center for Clinical Bioethics, GUMC; Chairman, President's Council on Bioethics
Pentecost, Michael J., M.D.	Chairman, Department of Radiology, GUMC (1996–2005); Director, Institute for Health Policy in Radiology, American College of Radiology, Reston VA; Chief of Radiology, Mid Atlantic Permanente Medical Group, Kaiser Permanente, Rockville, MD
Perloff, Joseph K., M.D.	Streisand/American Heart Association Professor of Medicine and Pediatrics, Emeritus; Founding Director, Ahmanson/UCLA Adult Congenital Heart Disease Center, University of California, Los Angeles
Perry, Robert G.	Trustee, GWU

Persily, Nancy A.	Various positions, GWUMC (1993–97); Assistant Provost and Associate Dean for Academic Affairs, University at Albany School of Public Health SUNY, Albany, NY
Piemme, Thomas E., M.D.	Chairman, Department of Health Care Sciences, GWUSM (1974–78); Director and Associate Dean, Office of Continuing Education, GWUMC (1978–98)
Pieper, Jay	VP, Corporate Development and Treasury Affairs, Partners HealthCare System Inc., Boston, MA
Pizzo, Philip A., M.D.	Dean, Stanford University School of Medicine, Stanford, CA
Porterfield, Daniel R., Ph.D.	VP for Public Affairs and Strategic Development, GU
Potter, John	Director, United States Military Cancer Institute of the Uniformed Services University of the Health Sciences, Bethesda, MD; Founding Director, Lombardi GUMC (1967–87)
Powell, Deborah E., M.D.	Dean, University of Minnesota Medical School and Assistant VP for Clinical Sciences, University of Minnesota, Minneapolis, MN
Prescott, John E., M.D.	Dean, West Virginia University School of Medicine, Morgantown, WV
Pyles, Brian T.	Associate VP for Finance and Planning, University of Toledo College of Medicine, Toledo, OH
Rackley, Charles E., M.D.	Chairman, Department of Medicine (1982–88); Professor of Medicine and Director, Lipid Disorder Center, GUMC
Ratner, Robert E., M.D.	VP for Scientific Affairs, MedStar Research Institute
Reiss, David, M.D.	Vivian Gill Distinguished Research Professor, Department of Psychiatry and Behavioral Sciences, GWUSM

Rennert, Owen M., M.D.	Chairman, Department of Pediatrics, GUMC (1988–98); Scientific Director, National Institute of Child Health and Human Development, National Institutes of Health, Bethesda, MD
Retchin, Sheldon M., M.D.	VP for Health Sciences, Virginia Commonwealth University; CEO, Virginia Commonwealth University Health System, Richmond, VA
Rich, Robert R., M.D.	Senior VP for Medicine, University of Alabama at Birmingham and Dean, University of Alabama School of Medicine, Birmingham, AL
Richardson, Mark A., M.D.	Dean, University of Oregon School of Medicine, Portland, OR
Richardson, William C., Ph.D.	President Emeritus, Johns Hopkins University; President Emeritus, W.K. Kellogg Foundation.
Richert, John R., M.D.	Chairman, Department of Microbiology and Immunology, GUMC (1997–2005); VP, Research and Clinical Programs, National Multiple Sclerosis Society, New York, NY
Rickles, Frederick R., M.D.	Professor of Medicine and Pediatrics, GWUSM; Associate VP for Health Research, Compliance and Technology Transfer, GWUMC (1998–2003); CEO and Executive Director, The Federation of Societies for Experimental Biology (FASEB), Bethesda, MD
Robillard, Jean E., M.D.	Dean, University of Iowa Roy J. and Lucille A. Carver College of Medicine, Iowa City, IA
Robinowitz, Carolyn B., M.D.	Clinical Professor of Psychiatry and Behavioral Science, GWSM; Clinical Professor of Psychiatry, GTMC

Rogers, Mark C., M.D.

Principal and Managing Director, Bradmer Ventures, Fisher Island, FL; Clinical Professor of Anesthesiology, Critical Care Medicine, and Pediatrics, Johns Hopkins University School of Medicine

Rosenberg, Joel, M.D.

Clinical Professor of Medicine, GWUSM; Director of Clinical Cardiology, GWUH

Rosenblatt, Michael, M.D.

Dean, Tufts University School of Medicine, Boston, MA

Ross, Arthur J., III, M.D.

Dean, Chicago Medical School, North Chicago, IL

Roth, Paul, M.D.

Dean, University of New Mexico School of Medicine, Albuquerque, NM

Rothman, Judith

Associate Vice Chancellor, Finance and Senior Associate Dean, Finance and Administration, University of California, Los Angeles School of Medicine, Los Angeles, CA

Rubenstein, Arthur H., M.B., B.Ch.

Dean, University of Pennsylvania School of Medicine and EVP, University of Pennsylvania for the Health System, Philadelphia, PA

Samet, Kenneth A.

President and COO, MedStar

Sandlow, Leslie J., M.D.

Senior Associate Dean for Educational Affairs, University of Illinois at Chicago College of Medicine, Chicago, IL

Sansing, Susan R.

Business Manager, University of South Alabama College of Medicine, Mobile, AL

Schaengold, Phillip S., J.D.

CEO and Managing Director, GWUH (1997–2000); CEO, University Hospital; Senior VP for Hospital Affairs, SUNY Upstate Medical University, Syracuse, NY

Scheinman, Steven, M.D. — Senior VP and Dean, College of Medicine, SUNY Upstate Medical University, Syracuse, NY

Schimpff, Stephen C., M.D. — Professor of Medicine, University of Maryland School of Medicine; EVP and COO, University of Maryland Medical System (1985–99); CEO, University of Maryland Medical Center (1999–2004)

Schlegel, C. Richard, M.D., Ph.D. — Chairman, Department of Pathology, GUMC

Schroeder, James L., M.D. — President and CEO, Northwestern Medical Faculty Foundation, Feinberg School of Medicine, Northwestern University, Chicago, IL

Schroeder, Stephen A., M.D. — Distinguished Professor of Health and Health Care, Department of Medicine, University of California, San Francisco

Schroth, Keith G. — Associate Dean of Fiscal Affairs, Louisiana State University School of Medicine, New Orleans, LA

Schwab, Steve J., M.D. — Executive Dean, University of Tennessee College of Medicine, Memphis, TN

Schwind, Ann — Associate Dean and CFO, Division of the Biological Sciences, Pritzker School of Medicine, University of Chicago, Chicago, IL

Scott, James L., M.D — Dean, GWUSM

Seides, Stuart F., M.D. — Clinical Professor of Medicine, Division of Cardiology, GWUSM; Board of Directors, WHC

Sekhar, Laligam N., M.D. — Professor and Chairman, Department of Neurological Surgery, GWUMC (1993–99); Professor and Vice Chairman, Department of Neurological Surgery, University of Washington School of Medicine, Seattle, WA

Seneff, Michael G., M.D.

Director, Intensive Care Units, GWUH

Shalala, Donna E., Ph.D.

President, University of Miami, Miami, FL

Shesser, Robert F., M.D.

Chairman, Department of Emergency Medicine, GWUSM

Silber, John R., Ph.D.

President Emeritus, Boston University, Boston, MA

Silva, Carlos A., M.D.

Medical Director, GWUH

Simon, David B., M.D.

Clinical Professor of Medicine, GWUSM

Simon, Gary L., M.D., Ph.D.

Director, Division of Infectious Diseases, Department of Medicine, GWUSM

Siwek, Jay, M.D.

Chairman, Department of Family Medicine, GUMC

Smith, Mark S., M.D.

Chairman, Departments of Emergency Medicine, GUMC and WHC

Solomon, Allen, M.D.

Director, Cardiac Arrhythmia Service, GUMC (2000–2004); Professor of Medicine, GWSM and Director, Coronary Care Unit, GWUH

Souba, Wiley W., M.D., Sc.D.

Dean, Ohio State University School of Medicine, Columbus, OH

Sousa, Aron, M.D.

Acting Associate Dean for Academic Affairs, College of Human Medicine, Michigan State University, East Lansing, MI

Spielberg, Stephen P., M.D., Ph.D.

Dean, Dartmouth Medical School and VP for Health Affairs, Dartmouth College, Hanover, NH

Spies, James B., M.D.

Chairman, Department of Radiology, GUMC

Stapleton, John, M.D.

Professor of Medicine Emeritus; Medical Director, GUH (1967–88)

Storey-Johnson, Carol L., M.D.

Senior Associate Dean (Education), Weill Medical College of Cornell University, New York, NY

Strada, Samuel, Ph.D.

Interim Dean and Senior Associate Dean for Basic Sciences, University of South Alabama College of Medicine, Mobile, AL

Stromberg, Clifford D., J.D.

Partner, Hogan & Hartson

Swearingen, Christine W.

Senior VP, Strategic Planning, MedStar

Taylor, Robert E., M.D., Ph.D.

Interim Dean, Howard University College of Medicine, Washington, DC

Thibault, George E., M.D.

VP, Clinical Affairs, Partners HealthCare System, Inc., Boston, MA

Thomas, William L., M.D

EVP, Medical Affairs, MedStar

Tisher, C. Craig, M.D.

Dean, University of Florida College of Medicine, Gainesville, FL

Trachtenberg, Stephen Joel

President, GWU

Vander Hoek, Michael

Interim Director, Lombardi, GUMCO

Verbalis, Joseph G., M.D.

Interim Chairman, Department of Medicine, GUMC

Verdile, Vincent P., M.D.

Dean and EVP for Health Affairs, Albany Medical College, Albany, NY

Waldhorn, Richard E., M.D.

Chairman, Department of Medicine, GUMC (2002–4); Senior Investigator, Center for Biosecurity, Baltimore, MD; Distinguished Scholar, University of Pittsburgh

Wallace, Robert B., M.D.

Chairman, Department of Surgery (1980–95) and Chief, Division of Cardiothoracic Surgery (1980–96), GUMC

Walsh, Raymond J., Ph.D.

Chairman, Department of Anatomy and Cell Biology, GWUSM

Wartofsky, Leonard, M.D.

Chairman, Department of Medicine, WHC; Professor of Medicine, GUMC

Wasserman, Alan G., M.D.

Chairman, Department of Medicine, GWUSM; President and Chairman of the Board of Trustees, MFA

Weglicki, William B., M.D.	Professor of Medicine and Physiology; Director, Division of Physiology and Experimental Medicine, Department of Medicine, GWUSM
Weingold, Allan B., M.D.	Professor Emeritus of Obstetrics and Gynecology, GWUSM
Werner, Leonard S., M.D.	Associate Dean for Medical Education, Loma Linda University School of Medicine, Loma Linda, CA
Wesnousky, Katherine A.	Controller, University of California–Davis Health System, Davis, CA
Whelton, Paul K., M.D.	Dean, Tulane University School of Medicine and Senior VP for Health Sciences, Tulane University Health Sciences Center, New Orleans, LA
Wiesel, Sam W., M.D.	Chairman, Department of Orthopedic Surgery, GUMC; EVP, Health Sciences and Executive Dean, GUMC (1996–2002); Senior VP GU and Dean of Clinical Affairs, GUMC (2002–3)
Wilcox, Christopher S., M.D., Ph.D.	Chief, Division of Nephrology and Hypertension, Department of Medicine, GUMC
Wildenthal, Kern, M.D., Ph.D.	President, University of Texas Southwestern Medical Center at Dallas, Dallas, TX
Williams, John F., Jr., M.D.	Provost, GWU; VP for Health Affairs, GWUMC
Winchester, James F., M.D.	Professor of Medicine, GUMC (1987–2000); Professor of Clinical Medicine, Albert Einstein College of Medicine of Yeshiva University, Bronx, NY
Woosley, Raymond L., M.D., Ph.D.	Chairman, Department of Pharmacology, GUMC (1988–2000); President and CEO, The C-Path Institute, Phoenix, AZ
Worth, Michael J.	Professor of Non-Profit Management, GWU

Wyatt, Lisa	Senior VP, Public Affairs and Marketing, WHC; VP, Marketing/MedStar Health Washington region
Wynne, Joshua, M.D.	Executive Associate Dean, University of North Dakota School of Medicine and Health Sciences, Grand Forks, ND
Zager, Laurie, R.N.	Administrative Director, Cardiovascular Research Institute, MedStar
Zeglis, John D.	Emeritus Trustee, GWU; CEO (retired), AT&T Wireless Group, Culver, IN
Ziskind, Andrew A., M.D.	President, Barnes-Jewish Hospital, St. Louis, MO

Notes

Preface

1. Kastor, JA. *Mergers of Teaching Hospitals in Boston, New York, and Northern California.* Ann Arbor: University of Michigan Press, 2001.
2. Kastor, JA. *Governance of Teaching Hospitals: Turmoil at Penn and Hopkins.* Baltimore: Johns Hopkins University Press, 2004.
3. Kastor, JA. *Specialty Care in the Era of Managed Care: Cleveland Clinic versus University Hospital of Cleveland.* Baltimore: Johns Hopkins University Press, 2005.

ONE: Washington and Its Academic Medical Centers

1. LaRosa, John C., M.D., Brooklyn, NY, by telephone 3/24/05.
2. Chapman, Thomas W., Ed.D., Washington, DC, 11/11/05.
3. Schaengold, Phillip S., J.D., Syracuse, NY, by telephone 1/6/06.
4. LaRosa, John C., M.D., Brooklyn, NY, by e-mail 11/7/06.
5. Shesser, Robert F., M.D., Washington, DC, 7/15/05.
6. McLean, Daniel P., McAllen, TX, by telephone 11/10/05.
7. Pawlson, L. Gregory, M.D., Washington, DC, by telephone 3/21/05.
8. Bowles, L. Thompson, M.D., Chevy Chase, MD, by telephone 3/21/05.
9. Greenberg, Warren, Ph.D., Washington, DC, by telephone 3/24/05.
10. Woosley, Raymond L., M.D., Ph.D., Tucson, AZ, by telephone 4/5/06.
11. Williams, John F., Jr., M.D., Washington, DC, 3/30/05.
12. Goldstein, Allan L., Ph.D., Washington, DC, 9/2/05.

TWO: George Washington University: Selling the Hospital

1. Trachtenberg, Stephen J., J.D., Washington, DC, 6/19/06.
2. Blumenthal D, Weissman JS. Selling Teaching Hospitals to Investor-owned Hospital Chains: Three Case Studies. *Health Affairs* 2000;19:158–166.
3. Katz, Louis H., Washington, DC, 12/19/05.
4. Trachtenberg, Stephen J. "Darwin Goes to Medical School or the Survival of the Academic Medical Center," 4/17/02.
5. Williams, John F., Jr., M.D., Washington, DC, 2/28/06.
6. "If You Can't Beat Em . . ." *Modern Healthcare,* 4/3/06.
7. Schaengold, Phillip S., J.D., Syracuse, NY, by telephone 1/6/06.
8. Weingold, Allan B., M.D., Washington, DC, by telephone 1/5/06.
9. Moxley, John H., III, M.D., Los Angeles, CA, by telephone 10/4/05.

10. Weingold, Allan B., M.D., Washington, DC, by telephone 6/24/05.

11. Birnbaum, Philip S., Washington, DC, 3/25/05.

12. Rogers, Mark C., M.D., New York, NY, by telephone 4/29/05.

13. McLean, Daniel P., McAllen, TX, by telephone 11/10/05.

14. Williams, John F., Jr., M.D., Washington, DC, 3/30/05.

15. Smith, Mark S., M.D., Washington, DC, by telephone 1/25/06.

16. Meyer, Roger E., M.D., Bethesda, MD, by e-mail 1/9/06.

17. Neviaser, Robert J., M.D., Washington, DC, 12/1/05.

18. Larsen, John W., M.D., Washington, DC, 9/16/05.

19. Seneff, Michael G., M.D., Washington, DC, 9/28/05.

20. Larsen, John W., M.D., Washington, DC, by e-mail 1/6/06.

21. Ghezzi, Keith T., M.D., Owings Mills, MD, 7/12/05.

22. Katz, Louis H., Washington, DC, 9/23/05.

23. Stephen J. Trachtenberg. "GWU Appropriation—Open and Honest." *The Washington Post*, 3/12/92.

24. Pawlson, L. Gregory, M.D., Washington, DC, by telephone 3/21/05.

25. Amy Goldstein. "Frustrations Cited as GWU Officials Quit." *The Washington Post*, 2/21/92.

26. Zeglis, John D., J.D., Culver, IN, by telephone 12/9/05.

27. Kastor, JA. New York—Presbyterian: Formation. In: *Mergers of Teaching Hospitals in Boston, New York, and Northern California.* Ann Arbor: University of Michigan Press, 2001, chap. 4, 125–126.

28. Elting, Jeffrey A., M.D., Washington, DC, by telephone 11/17/05.

29. Jarrett, Thomas W., M.D., Baltimore, MD, by telephone 1/17/06.

30. Trachtenberg, Stephen J., J.D., Washington, DC, 9/2/05.

31. Brand, Joseph L., J.D., Washington, DC, 11/21/05.

32. Chapman, Thomas W., Ed.D., Washington, DC, 11/11/05.

33. Barch, Michael M., Washington, DC, by telephone 3/10/05.

34. Cohen, Sheldon S., J.D., Washington, DC, 10/6/05.

35. Schaengold, Phillip S., J.D., Syracuse, NY, by e-mail 1/12/06.

36. Perry, Robert G., Washington, DC, 11/3/05.

37. Clough, E. Craig, Lexington, KY, by telephone 3/1/05.

38. Loop, Floyd D., M.D., Cleveland, OH, by telephone 1/10/06.

39. Cosgrove, Delos, M.D., Cleveland, OH, by telephone 8/4/06.

40. O'Leary, Dennis S., M.D., Chicago, IL, by telephone 4/21/05.

41. Shesser, Robert F., M.D., Washington, DC, 7/15/05.

42. Carr, Oliver T., Jr., J.D., Washington, DC, 12/5/05.

43. Hochberg, Mark S., M.D., New York, NY, by telephone 1/13/06.

44. Bowles, L. Thompson, M.D., Chevy Chase, MD, by telephone 3/21/05.

45. Manatt, Charles T., J.D., Washington, DC, 12/1/05.

46. Gurne, Patricia D., J.D., Washington, DC, 12/12/05.

47. Stromberg, Clifford D., J.D., Washington, DC, by telephone 6/16/06.

48. Jonathan Gardner. "CON Law Sparks Battle between Institutions." *Modern Health Care*, 2/19/96.

49. Stuart Auerbach. "Another Suitor for GW Hospital; Medlantic Is Latest to Bid for University's Facility." *The Washington Post*, 10/18/96.

50. Jonathan Gardner. "Still More Scrutiny: District of Columbia Legislation Would Add Obstacles to For-profit Deals." *Modern Health Care*, 3/24/97.

51. Amy Goldstein, Hamil R. Harris. "GWU Escapes Proposed Limits on Sales of Non-profit Hospitals." *The Washington Post*, 6/4/97.

52. Chiappinelli, Vincent A., Ph.D., Washington, DC, 4/4/05.

53. Katz, Richard J., M.D., Washington, DC, 3/30/05.

54. Amy Goldstein. "Tenn. Firm to Take over GWU Hospital." *The Washington Post*, 10/26/96.

55. Miller, Alan B., King of Prussia, PA, 9/19/05.

56. Amy Goldstein. "GWU to Sell Hospital to Health Chain; Large For-profit Firm Will Pay $125 Million." *The Washington Post*, 4/4/97.

57. Jonathan Gardner. "Tenet Rival Nabs Deal with GWU." *Modern Health Care*, 4/7/97.

58. Karcher, Donald S., M.D., Washington, DC, 9/2/05.

59. Amy Goldstein. "Sale of GWU Hospital Stirs Relief, Uncertainty; Workers Worry about Level of New Investment." *The Washington Post*, 5/5/97.

60. Jonathan Gardner. "GWU Hospital, Exempt from New D.C. Law, Does For-profit via Deal." *Modern Health Care*, 8/4/97.

61. Schaengold, Phillip S., J.D., Syracuse, NY, by telephone 1/6/06.

62. David S. Hilzenrath. "GWU Plans to Build New Hospital; Officials Cite Need for Modern Facility." *The Washington Post*, 2/26/98.

63. Jonathan Gardner. "On the Rebound: GWU Hospital Realizes Benefits of Investor Ownership." *Modern Health Care*, 8/10/99.

64. Silva, Carlos A., M.D., Washington, DC, 8/31/05.

65. Akman, Jeffrey S., M.D., Washington, DC, 8/31/05.

66. Berrigan, Michael J., M.D., Ph.D., Washington, DC, by telephone 9/8/05.

67. El-Bayoumi, Jehan, M.D., Washington, DC, 9/16/05.

68. Faselis, Charles J., M.D., Washington, DC, by telephone 8/1/05.

69. Goldstein, Allan L., Ph.D., Washington, DC, 9/2/05.

70. Mrazek, David A., M.D., Rochester, MN, by telephone 8/9/05.

71. Walsh, Raymond J., Ph.D., Washington, DC, 5/25/05.

72. Weglicki, William B., M.D., Washington, DC, 7/15/05.

73. Amsterdam, Philip S., West Orange, NJ, by telephone 12/22/05.

74. Curzon, Myron P., J.D., Bethesda, MD, 11/21/05.

75. Irani, Sands K., M.D., Chevy Chase, MD, by telephone 8/25/05.

76. Manyak, Michael J., M.D., Princeton, NJ, 7/25/05.

77. Simon, Gary L., M.D., Ph.D., Washington, DC, 3/25/05.

78. Barnhill, Raymond L., M.D., Miami, FL, by telephone 7/26/05.

79. Reiss, David, M.D., Washington, DC, 9/27/05.

80. Reiss, David, M.D., Washington, DC, by e-mail 1/15/06.

THREE: George Washington University: Separating the Practice Plan

1. Hastings, Douglas A., J.D., Washington, DC, 11/22/05.

2. Katz, Louis H., Washington, DC, 12/19/05.

3. Faselis, Charles J., M.D., Washington, DC, by telephone 8/1/05.

4. Wasserman, Alan G., M.D., Washington, DC, 4/4/05.
5. Jarrett, Thomas W., M.D., Baltimore, MD, by telephone 1/17/06.
6. Larsen, John W., M.D., Washington, DC, 9/16/05.
7. Brand, Joseph L., J.D., Washington, DC, 11/21/05.
8. Williams, John F., Jr., M.D., Washington, DC, 2/28/06.
9. Elliott, Lloyd H., Ed.D., Washington, DC, by telephone 11/11/05
10. Cohen, Sheldon S., J.D., Washington, DC, 10/6/05.
11. Bass, Gerald H., Washington, DC, 4/4/05.
12. Bass, Gerald H., Washington, DC, 2/28/06.
13. Smith, Mark S., M.D., Washington, DC, by telephone 1/25/06.
14. Sekhar, Laligam N., M.D., Seattle, WA, by telephone 11/17/05.
15. Zeglis, John D., J.D., Culver, IN, by telephone 12/9/05.
16. Curzon, Myron P., J.D., Bethesda, MD, 11/21/05.
17. Perry, Robert G., Washington, DC, 11/3/05.
18. Pawlson, L. Gregory, M.D., Washington, DC, by telephone 3/21/05.
19. Simon, Gary L., M.D., Ph.D., Washington, DC, 3/25/05.
20. Goldstein, Allan L., Ph.D., Washington, DC, 9/2/05.
21. Katz, Louis H., Washington, DC, 9/23/05.
22. Williams, John F., Jr., M.D., Washington, DC, 3/30/05.
23. Trachtenberg, Stephen J. "Darwin Goes to Medical School or the Survival of the Academic Medical Center." 4/17/02.
24. Shesser, Robert F., M.D., Washington, DC, 7/15/05.
25. Kelly, John J., M.D., Washington, DC, by e-mail 2/9/06.
26. Karcher, Donald S., M.D., Washington, DC, 9/2/05.
27. Manyak, Michael J., M.D., Princeton, NJ, 7/25/05.
28. Neviaser, Robert J., M.D., Washington, DC, 12/1/05.
29. Scott, James L., Washington, DC, 5/2/05.
30. Seneff, Michael G., M.D., Washington, DC, 9/28/05.
31. Weingold, Allan B., M.D., Washington, DC, by telephone 6/24/05.
32. Katz, Louis H., Washington, DC, 12/19/05.
33. Berrigan, Michael J., M.D., Ph.D., Washington, DC, by telephone 9/8/05.
34. Katz, Richard J., M.D., Washington, DC, 3/30/05.
35. Silva, Carlos A., M.D., Washington, DC, 8/31/05.
36. Irani, Sands K., M.D., Chevy Chase, MD, by telephone 8/25/05.
37. Giordano, Joseph M., M.D., Washington, DC, 5/2/05.
38. Schaengold, Phillip S., J.D., Syracuse, NY, by telephone 1/6/06.
39. Badger SL, Bosch RG, Toteja P. Rapid Implementation of an Electronic Health Record in an Academic Setting. *Journal of Healthcare Information Management* 2005;19:34–40.
40. Kelly, John J., M.D., Washington, DC, by e-mail 2/7/06.
41. Weglicki, William B., M.D., Washington, DC, 7/15/05.
42. Kelly, John J., M.D., Washington, DC, 9/16/05.
43. Akman, Jeffrey S., M.D., Washington, DC, 8/31/05.
44. Barnhill, Raymond L., M.D., Miami, FL, by telephone 7/26/05.
45. Berg, Patricia E., Ph.D., Washington, DC, 7/15/05.
46. McCaffrey, Timothy A., Ph.D., Washington, DC, 5/25/05.
47. Reiss, David, M.D., Washington, DC, 9/27/05.
48. Lehman, Donald R., Ph.D., Washington, DC, 9/23/05.

49. Lehman, Donald R., Ph.D., Washington, DC, by e-mail 12/28/05.
50. NIH Awards to Medical Schools by Rank. Fiscal Year 2004. Department of internal medicine. http://grants1.nih.gov/grants/award/rank/internal04.htm. 2005.
51. Kelly, John J., M.D., Washington, DC, by e-mail 3/2/06.
52. Rogers, Mark C., M.D., New York, NY, by telephone 4/29/05.
53. O'Leary, Dennis S., M.D., Chicago, IL, by telephone 4/21/05.
54. Birnbaum, Philip S., Washington, DC, 3/25/05.
55. LaRosa, John C., M.D., Brooklyn, NY, by telephone 3/24/05.
56. Schimpff, Stephen C., M.D., Baltimore, MD, 4/7/05.
57. McLean, Daniel P., McAllen, TX, by telephone 11/10/05.
58. Rosenberg, Joel, M.D., Washington, DC, 10/6/05.
59. Meyer, Roger E., M.D., Bethesda, MD, 3/28/05.
60. Leon, Martin B., M.D., New York, NY, by telephone 8/30/05.
61. Katz, Nevin M., M.D., Washington, DC, by telephone 2/14/06.
62. Adkins, Mark S., M.D., New York, NY, by telephone 12/15/05.
63. Lough, Frederick C., M.D., Washington, DC, 12/19/05.
64. Silva, Carlos A., M.D., Washington, DC, by e-mail 1/12/06.
65. Simon, David B., M.D., Washington, DC, 9/23/05.

FOUR: George Washington University: Closing the HMO

1. Piemme, Thomas E., M.D., Surprise, AZ, by telephone 8/29/05.
2. Ott, John E., M.D., Washington, DC, 3/11/05.
3. Pawlson, L. Gregory, M.D., Washington, DC, by telephone 3/21/05.
4. Ott, John E., M.D., Washington, DC, by e-mail 1/19/06.
5. Mullan, Fitzhugh, M.D., Washington, DC, by telephone 1/5/06.
6. Chaufournier, Roger L., Washington, DC, by telephone 8/24/05.
7. Bowles, L. Thompson, M.D., Chevy Chase, MD, by telephone 3/21/05.
8. Meyer, Roger E., M.D., Bethesda, MD, by telephone 2/25/05.
9. Katz, Richard J., M.D., Washington, DC, 3/30/05.
10. Barch, Michael M., Washington, DC, by telephone 3/10/05.
11. Ott, John E., M.D., Washington, DC, by telephone 2/7/06.
12. O'Leary, Dennis S., M.D., Chicago, IL, by telephone 4/21/05.
13. Pawlson, L. Gregory, M.D., Washington, DC, by e-mail 1/6/06.
14. Berrigan, Michael J., M.D., Ph.D., Washington, DC, by telephone 9/8/05.
15. Sekhar, Laligam N., M.D., Seattle, WA, by telephone 11/17/05.
16. Gardner, J. GWU does about-face on its HMO. www.modernhealthcare.com/article.cms?articleId=12541. 7/20/98.
17. Aronovitch, Stanley I., Ph.D., Phoenix, AZ, by telephone 7/22/05.
18. Zeglis, John D., J.D., Culver, IN, by telephone 12/9/05.
19. Persily, Nancy A., Albany, NY, by telephone 1/24/06.
20. Bass, Gerald H., Washington, DC, 4/4/05.
21. Williams, John F., Jr., M.D., Washington, DC, 3/30/05.
22. Brand, Joseph L., J.D., Washington, DC, 11/21/05.
23. Giordano, Joseph M., M.D., Washington, DC, 5/2/05.
24. Retchin, Sheldon M., M.D., Richmond, VA, by telephone 1/6/06.
25. Katz, Louis H., Washington, DC, 12/19/05.

FIVE: George Washington University and Its Medical School

1. Kayser, EL. *Bricks without Straw.* New York: Appleton-Century-Crofts, 1970.
2. Kayser, EL. *A Medical Center. The Institutional Development of Medical Education at George Washington University.* Washington, DC: George Washington University Press, 1973.
3. Association of American Medical Colleges. US medical school year of establishment. 2005.
4. The Corcoran Gallery of Art. www.corcoran.org/. 2006.
5. The Parrish Art Museum. www.parrishart.org/Current.asp?id=119. 2006.
6. Kayser, *A Medical Center,* 141.
7. Brady, Luther W., M.D., Philadelphia, PA, by telephone 12/14/05.
8. Kayser, *Bricks without Straw,* 217.
9. Kayser, *A Medical Center,* 165.
10. Birnbaum, Philip S., Washington, DC, 3/25/05.
11. O'Leary, Dennis S., M.D., Chicago, IL, by telephone 4/21/05.
12. Williams, John F., Jr., M.D., Washington, DC, 2/28/06.
13. Schimpff, Stephen C., M.D., Baltimore, MD, 4/7/05.
14. Meyer, Roger E., M.D., Bethesda, MD, 3/28/05.
15. Meyer, Roger E., M.D., Bethesda, MD, by telephone 2/25/05.
16. Trachtenberg, Stephen J., J.D., Washington, DC, 6/19/06.
17. Jonathan Gardner. "Executive Quits as School Considers Selling Hospital." *Modern Health Care,* 3/20/95.
18. Amy Goldstein. "GW Hospital Chief Quits in Dispute. Medical Center Faces Possible Sale, Merger." *The Washington Post,* 3/3/92.
19. John Lombardo. "Kaiser Ready to Buy GWU Health Plan." *Washington Business Journal,* 9/20/96.
20. Weingold, Allan B., M.D., Washington, DC, by telephone 6/24/05.
21. Ghezzi, Keith T., M.D., Owings Mills, MD, 7/12/05.
22. Trachtenberg, Stephen J., J.D., Washington, DC, 9/2/05.
23. Meyer, Roger E., M.D., Bethesda, MD, by telephone 12/27/05.
24. Sekhar, Laligam N., M.D., Seattle, WA, by e-mail 12/30/05.
25. Wasserman, Alan G., M.D., Washington, DC, by e-mail 4/5/05.
26. Wasserman, Alan G., M.D., Washington, DC, 4/4/05.
27. Brand, Joseph L., J.D., Washington, DC, 11/21/05.
28. Rickles, Frederick R., M.D., Bethesda, MD, by telephone 7/5/05.
29. Sekhar, Laligam N., M.D., Seattle, WA, by telephone 11/17/05.
30. Williams, John F., Jr., M.D., Washington, DC, 3/30/05.
31. Pawlson, L. Gregory, M.D., Washington, DC, by telephone 3/21/05.
32. Kastor, JA. University of Pennsylvania: After Kelley. In: *Governance of Teaching Hospitals: Turmoil at Penn and Hopkins.* Baltimore: Johns Hopkins University Press, 2004, chap. 5, 134–136.
33. Bass, Gerald H., Washington, DC, 4/4/05.
34. Manatt, Charles T., J.D., Washington, DC, 12/1/05.
35. Chiappinelli, Vincent A., Ph.D., Washington, DC, 4/4/05.
36. Karcher, Donald S., M.D., Washington, DC, 9/2/05.

37. Bass, Gerald H., Washington, DC, by e-mail 4/18/05.

38. Katz, Ruth J., Washington, DC, 4/11/05.

39. Berg, Patricia E., Ph.D., Washington, DC, 7/15/05.

40. Berg, Patricia E., Ph.D., Washington, DC, by e-mail 1/20/06.

41. Akman, Jeffrey S., M.D., Washington, DC, 8/31/05.

42. Manyak, Michael J., M.D., Princeton, NJ, 7/25/05.

43. Bowles, L. Thompson, M.D., Chevy Chase, MD, by telephone 3/21/05.

44. Scott, James L., Washington, DC, 5/2/05.

45. Reiss, David, M.D., Washington, DC, 9/27/05.

46. Katz, Louis H., Washington, DC, 9/23/05.

47. Amsterdam, Philip S., West Orange, NJ, by telephone 12/22/05.

48. NIH Awards to Medical Schools by Rank. Fiscal Year 2005. http://grants.nih.gov/grants/award/rank/medttl05.htm. 2006.

49. NIH Support to U.S. Medical Schools, FY's 1970–2000. http://grants1.nih.gov/grants/award/trends/medsup7000.txt. 3/15/01.

50. Association of American Medical Colleges. Number of Medical Schools with Students Enrolled. 2005.

51. Walsh, Raymond J., Ph.D., Washington, DC, 5/25/05.

52. Trachtenberg, Stephen J., J.D., Washington, DC, by e-mail 6/27/06.

53. Trachtenberg, Stephen J., J.D., Washington, DC, by letter 6/28/05.

54. Lazarus, Gerald S., M.D., Baltimore, MD, 11/8/05.

55. Batshaw, Mark L., M.D., Washington, DC, by telephone 8/8/05.

56. Giordano, Joseph M., M.D., Washington, DC, 5/2/05.

57. Hirshfield, Anne N., Ph.D., Washington, DC, 4/11/05.

58. McCaffrey, Timothy A., Ph.D., Washington, DC, 5/25/05.

59. Hotez, Peter J., M.D., Ph.D., Washington, DC, 5/26/05.

60. Katz, Richard J., M.D., Washington, DC, 3/30/05.

61. Larsen, John W., M.D., Washington, DC, 9/16/05.

62. Schroeder, Stephen A., M.D., San Francisco, CA, by telephone 3/23/05.

63. Simon, Gary L., M.D., Ph.D., Washington, DC, 3/25/05.

64. Weglicki, William B., M.D., Washington, DC, 7/15/05.

65. Shesser, Robert F., M.D., Washington, DC, 7/15/05.

66. Lehman, Donald R., Ph.D., Washington, DC, 9/23/05.

67. Goldstein, Allan L., Ph.D., Washington, DC, 9/2/05.

68. Faselis, Charles J., M.D., Washington, DC, by telephone 8/1/05.

69. Seneff, Michael G., M.D., Washington, DC, 9/28/05.

70. Weglicki, William B., M.D., Washington, DC, by e-mail 1/6/06.

71. Herzog, William R., Jr., M.D., Baltimore, MD, 8/23/05.

72. Kelly, John J., M.D., Washington, DC, 9/16/05.

73. Kastor, JA. Johns Hopkins University and Hospital: Unified Governance. In: *Governance of Teaching Hospitals: Turmoil at Penn and Hopkins*. Baltimore: Johns Hopkins University Press, 2004, chap. 7, 213–277.

74. Jarrett, Thomas W., M.D., Baltimore, MD, by telephone 1/17/06.

75. Adkins, Mark S., M.D., New York, NY, by telephone 12/15/05.

76. Reiss, David, M.D., Washington, DC, by e-mail 2/13/06.

77. Hotez, Peter J., M.D., Ph.D., Washington, DC, by e-mail 12/28/05.

78. Batshaw, Mark L., M.D., Washington, DC, by e-mail 11/2/05.

79. Batshaw, Mark L., M.D., Washington, DC, by e-mail 12/27/05.

80. Kastor, JA. University of Pennsylvania: Kelley the Builder. In: *Governance of Teaching Hospitals: Turmoil at Penn and Hopkins*. Baltimore: Johns Hopkins University Press, 2004, chap. 3, 52–54.

81. El-Bayoumi, Jehan, M.D., Washington, DC, 9/16/05.

82. Brosowsky, Jeremy M. The Unexpected Dr. Trachtenberg. *Washington Business Forward*. 2001;42.

83. Valerie Strauss. "GWU President Says He Will Step Down in 2007." *The Washington Post*, 4/5/06.

84. Stephen Joel Trachtenberg, President and Professor of Public Administration, The George Washington University. www.gwu.edu/gwpres/biography.html. 2005.

85. Carbonell, Nelson A., Jr., Reston, VA, 12/20/05.

86. Carr, Oliver T., Jr., J.D., Washington, DC, 12/5/05.

87. Chapman, Thomas W., Ed.D., Washington, DC, 11/11/05.

88. Chaufournier, Roger L., Washington, DC, by telephone 8/24/05.

89. Gurne, Patricia D., J.D., Washington, DC, 12/12/05.

90. Curzon, Myron P., J.D., Bethesda, MD, 11/21/05.

91. Greenberg, Warren, Ph.D., Washington, DC, by telephone 3/24/05.

92. Hochberg, Mark S., M.D., New York, NY, by telephone 1/13/06.

93. LaRosa, John C., M.D., Brooklyn, NY, by telephone 3/24/05.

94. Moxley, John H., III, M.D., Los Angeles, CA, by telephone 10/4/05.

95. Ott, John E., M.D., Washington, DC, 3/11/05.

96. Perry, Robert G., Washington, DC, 11/3/05.

97. Retchin, Sheldon M., M.D., Richmond, VA, by telephone 1/6/06.

98. Rogers, Mark C., M.D., New York, NY, by telephone 4/29/05.

99. Seides, Stuart F., M.D., Washington, DC, 6/29/05.

100. Shalala, Donna E., Ph.D., Miami, FL, by telephone 1/23/06.

101. Zeglis, John D., J.D., Culver, IN, by telephone 12/9/05.

102. Elliott, Lloyd H., Ed.D., Washington, DC, by telephone 11/11/05

103. Silber, John R., Ph.D., Boston, MA, by telephone 11/23/05.

104. Katz, Barrett, M.D., New York, NY, by telephone 7/13/05.

105. Trachtenberg, Stephen J. "Darwin Goes to Medical School or the Survival of the Academic Medical Center." 4/17/02.

106. College and university endowment funds 2005. www.nacubo.org/documents/about/FY05NESInstitutionsbyTotalAssets.pdf.

107. Worth, Michael J., Ph.D., Washington, DC, by telephone 6/28/06.

108. Price Jones, Laurel, Washington, DC, by e-mail 7/10/06.

109. Price Jones, Laurel, Washington, DC, by e-mail 7/31/06.

110. Martin Weil, Susan Kinzie. "Johns Hopkins Provost Chosen To Lead GWU." *The Washington Post*, 12/5/06.

111. Johns Hopkins University Provost Steven Knapp Selected As GW's 16th President. www.gwu.edu/%7Enewsctr/pressrelease.cfm?ann—id=24671. 2006.

SIX: Georgetown University: Selling the Hospital

1. Griffith, John F., M.D., Cincinnati, OH, by telephone 2/14/06.

2. Bondurant, Stuart, M.D., Washington, DC, 3/28/05.

3. Cavender, Laura, Washington, DC, by e-mail 9/28/06.

4. Cullen, Kevin J., M.D., Baltimore, MD, 6/27/05.

5. Porterfield, Daniel, Ph.D., Washington, DC, by telephone 9/15/06.

6. Katz, Paul, M.D., Miami, FL, by telephone 3/13/06.

7. Faden, Alan I., M.D., Washington, DC, by telephone 6/14/06.

8. Davis, F. Daniel, Ph.D., Washington, DC, by telephone 4/6/06.

9. Goldberg, Richard L., M.D., Washington, DC, by telephone 3/15/06.

10. Corn, Milton, M.D., Bethesda, MD, by telephone 4/7/06.

11. Jacobson, Robert J., M.B., B.Ch., West Palm Beach, FL, by telephone 6/1/06.

12. Lemp, Michael A., M.D., Washington, DC, by telephone 5/30/06.

13. Dym, Martin O., Ph.D., Potomac, MD, by telephone 6/26/06.

14. Cossman, Jeffrey, M.D., Seattle, WA, by telephone 9/11/06.

15. Kelly, Michael J., J.D., Ph.D., Baltimore, MD, 3/7/06.

16. Pearle, David L., M.D., Bethesda, MD, by telephone 4/4/06.

17. Wiesel, Sam W., M.D., Washington, DC, 1/26/06.

18. Rennert, Owen M., M.D., Bethesda, MD, by telephone 7/7/06.

19. Robinowitz, Carolyn, M.D., Washington, DC, by telephone 3/5/05.

20. Stapleton, John F., M.D., Arlington, VA, by telephone 5/30/06.

21. Milton Corn. https://ned.nih.gov/SrchDetail.asp?IndvUID=0010040179&ClickCount=1. 2006.

22. Bloem, Kenneth D., Elk Rapids, MI, by telephone 2/13/06.

23. O'Brien, Charles M., Jr., Pittsburgh, PA, by telephone 4/7/06.

24. Bloem, Kenneth D., Elk Rapids, MI, by telephone 2/20/06.

25. Pellegrino, Edmund D., M.D., Bethesda, MD, by telephone 6/23/06.

26. Bergin, Adrian G., Baltimore, MD, 7/17/06.

27. Cassem, Edwin H., M.D., Boston, MA, by telephone 6/3/06.

28. Ford, Nelson M., Washington, DC, by telephone 4/3/06.

29. Lippman, Marc E., M.D., Ann Arbor, MI, by telephone 3/16/06.

30. Jacobson, Robert J., M.B., B.Ch., West Palm Beach, FL, by e-mail 6/2/06.

31. Clauw, Daniel J., M.D., San Diego, CA, by telephone 6/26/06.

32. Cupples, Howard P., M.D., Annapolis, MD, by telephone 6/8/06.

33. Lumpkin, Michael D., Ph.D., Washington, DC, 2/9/06.

34. Flynn Hollander, Sharon, Washington, DC, by telephone 4/5/06.

35. Bondurant, Stuart, M.D., Washington, DC, by e-mail 3/5/07.

36. Campbell, Karen L., Grover Beach, CA, by telephone 7/6/06.

37. O'Brien, Charles M., Jr., Pittsburgh, PA, by e-mail 9/28/06.

38. DeGioia, John J., Ph.D., Washington, DC, 11/15/06.

39. Grossi, Richard A., Baltimore, MD, by mail 8/10/06.

40. Richert, John R., M.D., New York, NY, by telephone 4/19/06.

41. Haramati, Aviad, Ph.D., Baltimore, MD, 9/26/06.

42. Cerqueira, Manuel, M.D. Cleveland, OH, by telephone 6/27/05.

43. Seides, Stuart F., M.D., Washington, DC, 6/29/05.

44. Valerie Strauss. "Georgetown Moves to Replace Law Dean." *The Washington Post,* 4/9/98.

45. Valerie Strauss. "Law School Backers Blast GU." *The Washington Post,* 4/10/98.

46. Valerie Strauss. "A Rebellion at Georgetown Law." *The Washington Post,* 4/16/98.

47. Valerie Strauss. "Georgetown Decides to Retain Law Dean." *The Washington Post,* 4/18/98.

48. Georgetown University provost. http://provost.georgetown.edu. 2006.

49. Georgetown University administration. www.georgetown.edu/home/administra
tion.html. 2006.

50. Kelly, Michael J., J.D., Ph.D., Baltimore, MD, by telephone 11/17/06.

51. "Georgetown Vice President Resigns." *The Washington Post*, 8/30/98.

52. Caryle Murphy. "Georgetown President to Leave Next Year; Before Departing,
O'Donovan to Focus on Fund-raising Drive, Hospital Sale." *The Washington Post*, 3/21/00.

53. O'Boyle, Michael P., Cleveland, OH, by telephone 6/27/06.

54. Woosley, Raymond L., M.D., Ph.D., Tucson, AZ, by telephone 4/5/06.

55. Pentecost, Michael J., M.D., Rockville, MD, by telephone 6/28/06.

56. Verbalis, Joseph G., M.D., Washington, DC, 1/26/06.

57. Wilcox, Christopher S., M.D., Ph.D., Washington, DC, by telephone 6/14/06.

58. Cavender, Laura, Washington, DC, by e-mail 1/22/07.

59. College and university endowment funds 1999. http://chronicle.com/weekly/
v46/i24/stats/4624endowments.htm.

60. College and university endowment funds 2005. www.nacubo.org/documents/
about/FY05NESInstitutionsbyTotalAssets.pdf.

61. Faden, Alan I., M.D., Washington, DC, by telephone 6/21/06.

62. Carbonell, Nelson A., Jr., Reston, VA, 12/20/05.

63. Miller, Edward D., M.D., Baltimore, MD, 4/22/05.

64. Cavender, Laura, Washington, DC, by e-mail 1/22/07.

65. Cox, James L., M.D., Naples, FL, by telephone 5/24/06.

66. Report on GU's partnership with MedStar. 2002.

67. Drass, M. Joy, M.D., Washington, DC, 1/26/06.

68. Marzano, John A., Columbia, MD, by e-mail 1/25/07.

69. Alcorn, Karen, Washington, DC, by telephone 2/22/07.

70. Nelson, David B., M.D., Washington, DC, by telephone 7/7/06.

71. Drass, M. Joy, M.D., Washington, DC, by telephone 10/3/06.

72. Mitchell, Stephen Ray, M.D., Washington, DC, by telephone 7/10/06.

73. Brown, Ronald A., Baltimore, MD, 7/6/05.

74. Lynch, John H., M.D., Washington, DC, by telephone 8/31/06.

75. Waldhorn, Richard E., M.D., Baltimore, MD, by telephone 2/10/06.

76. Drass, M. Joy, M.D., Washington, DC, by e-mail 1/25/07.

77. Anderson, Minor W., Miami, FL, by telephone 6/1/06.

78. Lustbader, Jay M., M.D., Washington, DC, by telephone 9/11/06.

79. Siwek, Jay, M.D., Washington, DC, by telephone 8/29/06.

80. Vander Hoek, Michael P., Washington, DC, by telephone 6/28/06.

81. Corso, Paul J., M.D., Washington, DC, by telephone 8/1/06.

82. Kim, Young, M.D., Washington, DC, by telephone 8/9/06.

83. Schlegel, Richard, M.D., Ph.D., Washington, DC, by telephone 7/18/06.

84. Martuza, Robert L., M.D., Boston, MA, by telephone 7/17/06.

85. McDaniel, John P., Columbia, MD, by e-mail 3/14/06.

86. Meador, Kimford J., M.D., Gainesville, FL, by telephone 6/21/06.

87. Shumacker, HB, Jr. *The Evolution of Cardiac Surgery*. Bloomington: Indiana University Press, 2006, 212–213.

88. Kent, Kenneth M., M.D., Ph.D., Washington, DC.

89. Morad, Martin, Ph.D., Washington, DC, by telephone 4/15/06.

90. Perloff, Joseph K., M.D., Los Angeles, CA, by telephone 9/20/06.

91. Wallace, Robert B., M.D., McLean, VA, by telephone 5/26/06.

92. Gersh, Bernard J., M.B., B.Ch., Ph.D., Rochester, MN, by telephone 12/15/05.

93. Kastor, JA. Cleveland Clinic: The Clinical Factory. In: *Specialty Care in the Era of Managed Care: Cleveland Clinic versus University Hospital of Cleveland.* Baltimore: Johns Hopkins University Press, 2005, chap. 2, 61–71.

94. Rackley, Charles E., M.D., Washington, DC, by telephone 5/24/06.

95. Wartofsky, Leonard, M.D., Washington, DC, by telephone 7/20/06.

96. Samet, Kenneth A., Columbia, MD, 7/13/05.

97. Nelson, David B., M.D., Washington, DC, by e-mail 7/17/06.

98. Solomon, Allen J., M.D., Washington, DC, 5/2/05.

99. Pearle, David L., M.D., Bethesda, MD, by e-mail 10/3/06.

100. Miller, Leslie W., M.D., Washington, DC, by e-mail 10/2/06.

101. Nauta, Russell J., M.D., Cambridge, MA, by e-mail 10/19/06.

102. Evans, Stephen R. T., M.D., Washington, DC, by telephone 6/13/06.

103. Evans, Stephen R. T., M.D., Washington, DC, by e-mail 6/22/06.

104. Katz, Richard J., M.D., Washington, DC, 3/30/05.

105. Williams, John F., Jr., M.D., Washington, DC, 3/30/05.

106. Smith, Mark S., M.D., Washington, DC, by telephone 8/18/06.

107. Miller, Alan B., King of Prussia, PA, 9/19/05.

108. Wiesel, Sam W., M.D., Washington, DC, by e-mail 3/16/06.

109. McDaniel, John P., Columbia, MD, 7/13/05.

110. Diamond, Louis H., Rockville, MD, by telephone 6/8/06.

111. Kastor, JA. University of Pennsylvania: Kelley the Builder. In: *Governance of Teaching Hospitals: Turmoil at Penn and Hopkins.* Baltimore: Johns Hopkins University Press, 2004, chap. 3, 49–52.

112. Providence Hospital. www.provhosp.org/history—&—mission.htm. 2006.

113. Kastor, JA. University of Pennsylvania: After Kelley. In: *Governance of Teaching Hospitals: Turmoil at Penn and Hopkins.* Baltimore: Johns Hopkins University Press, 2004, chap. 5, 134–136.

SEVEN: Georgetown University: Selling the Practice Plan

1. O'Brien, Charles M., Jr., Pittsburgh, PA, by telephone 4/7/06.

2. Bergin, Adrian G., Baltimore, MD, 7/17/06.

3. Goldberg, Richard L., M.D., Washington, DC, by telephone 3/15/06.

4. Kent, Kenneth M., M.D., Ph.D., Washington, DC.

5. Davis, F. Daniel, Ph.D., Washington, DC, by telephone 4/6/06.

6. Mitchell, Stephen Ray, M.D., Washington, DC, by telephone 7/10/06.

7. Goldberg, Richard L., M.D., Washington, DC, by telephone 3/23/06.

8. Wiesel, Sam W., M.D., Washington, DC, by telephone 10/5/06.

9. Anderson, Minor W., Miami, FL, by telephone 6/1/06.

10. Curran, Michael J., Columbia, MD, 6/6/05.

11. Drass, M. Joy, M.D., Washington, DC, 1/26/06.

12. Ford, Nelson M., Washington, DC, by telephone 4/3/06.

13. Clauw, Daniel J., M.D., San Diego, CA, by telephone 6/26/06.

14. O'Boyle, Michael P., Cleveland, OH, by telephone 6/27/06.

15. Swearingen, Christine M., Columbia, MD, by telephone 6/12/06.

16. Bloem, Kenneth D., Elk Rapids, MI, by telephone 2/20/06.
17. Gioia, John J., Ph.D., Washington, DC, 11/15/06.
18. Goldberg, Richard L., M.D., Washington, DC, by e-mail 9/30/06.
19. Haramati, Aviad, Ph.D., Baltimore, MD, 9/26/06.
20. Report on GU's partnership with MedStar. 2002.
21. Brown, Ronald A., Baltimore, MD, 7/6/05.
22. Epstein, Steven A., M.D., Washington, DC, by telephone 3/31/06.
23. Cerqueira, Manuel, M.D., Cleveland, OH, by telephone 6/27/05.
24. Campbell, Karen L., Grover Beach, CA, by telephone 7/6/06.
25. Waldhorn, Richard E., M.D., Baltimore, MD, by telephone 2/10/06.
26. Marzano, John A., Columbia, MD, by e-mail 1/25/07.
27. Robinowitz, Carolyn, M.D., Washington, DC, by telephone 3/5/05.
28. Wiesel, Sam W., M.D., Washington, DC, 1/26/06.
29. Katz, Paul, M.D., Miami, FL, by telephone 3/13/06.
30. Pearle, David L., M.D., Bethesda, MD, by telephone 4/4/06.
31. Woosley, Raymond L., M.D., Ph.D., Tucson, AZ, by telephone 4/5/06.
32. Katz, Nevin M., M.D., Washington, DC, by telephone 2/14/06.
33. Nevin M. Katz, M.D., Appellant v. Georgetown University, et al., Appellees. www
.ll.georgetown.edu/federal/judicial/dc/opinions/00opinions/00-7265a.html. 2001.
34. Pentecost, Michael J., M.D., Rockville, MD, by telephone 6/28/06.
35. Pentecost, Michael J., M.D., Rockville, MD, by telephone 7/21/06.
36. Davidson, Bruce J., M.D., Washington, DC, by telephone 6/15/06.
37. Winchester, James F., M.D., New York, NY, by telephone 7/5/06.
38. Cupples, Howard P., M.D., Annapolis, MD, by telephone 6/8/06.
39. Kim, Young, M.D., Washington, DC, by telephone 8/9/06.
40. Lustbader, Jay M., M.D., Washington, DC, by telephone 9/11/06.
41. Lynch, John H., M.D., Washington, DC, by telephone 8/31/06.
42. Siwek, Jay, M.D., Washington, DC, by telephone 8/29/06.
43. Wiesel, Sam W., M.D., Washington, DC, by telephone 9/1/06.
44. Cavender, Laura, Washington, DC, by e-mail 1/22/07.
45. Faden, Alan I., M.D., Washington, DC, by telephone 6/21/06.
46. Bondurant, Stuart, M.D., Washington, DC, 3/28/05.
47. Corso, Paul J., M.D., Washington, DC, by telephone 8/1/06.
48. Richert, John R., M.D., New York, NY, by telephone 4/19/06.
49. Wilcox, Christopher S., M.D., Ph.D., Washington, DC, by telephone 6/14/06.
50. Kelly, Michael J., J.D. Ph.D., Baltimore, MD, 3/7/06.
51. Cullen, Kevin J., M.D., Baltimore, MD, 6/27/05.
52. Faden, Alan I., M.D., Washington, DC, by telephone 6/14/06.
53. Lumpkin, Michael D., Ph.D., Washington, DC, 2/9/06.
54. Martuza, Robert L., M.D., Boston, MA, by telephone 7/17/06.
55. Rennert, Owen M., M.D., Bethesda, MD, by telephone 7/7/06.
56. Bloem, Kenneth D., Elk Rapids, MI, by telephone 2/13/06.
57. Meador, Kimford J., M.D., Gainesville, FL, by telephone 6/21/06.
58. Evans, Stephen R. T., M.D., Washington, DC, by telephone 6/13/06.
59. Healton, Edward B., M.D., Washington, DC, by telephone 8/16/06.
60. Nelson, David B., M.D., Washington, DC, by telephone 7/7/06.
61. Lippman, Marc E., M.D., Ann Arbor, MI, by telephone 3/16/06.

62. Corn, Milton, M.D., Bethesda, MD, by telephone 4/7/06.
63. Potter, John F., M.D., Washington, DC, by telephone 2/10/05.
64. Dretchen, Kenneth L., Ph.D., Washington, DC, 2/9/06.
65. Milton Corn. https://ned.nih.gov/SrchDetail.asp?IndvUID=0010040179&Click Count=1. 2006.
66. Bondurant, Stuart, M.D., Washington, DC, by e-mail 1/23/07.
67. Cossman, Jeffrey, M.D., Seattle, WA, by telephone 9/11/06.
68. Mitchell, Stephen Ray, M.D., Washington, DC, by e-mail 1/22/07.
69. Mitchell, Stephen Ray, M.D., Washington, DC, by e-mail 7/18/06.
70. Spies, James B., M.D., Washington, DC, by telephone 7/14/06.
71. Goldberg, Richard L., M.D., Washington, DC, by telephone 6/8/06.
72. Stapleton, JF. *Upward Journey: The Story of Internal Medicine at Georgetown 1851–1981*. Washington, DC: Georgetown University, 1996.
73. "John Eisenberg Dies." *The Washington Post*, 3/11/02.
74. Verbalis, Joseph G., M.D., Washington, DC, 1/26/06.
75. Wiesel, Sam W., M.D., Washington, DC, by telephone 7/7/06.
76. Drass, M. Joy, M.D., Washington, DC, by e-mail 1/25/07.
77. Schlegel, Richard, M.D., Ph.D., Washington, DC, by telephone 7/18/06.
78. Dritschilo, Anatoly, M.D., Washington, DC, by telephone 5/25/06.
79. Bondurant, Stuart, M.D., Washington, DC, by e-mail 3/5/07.
80. Kastor, JA. *Mergers of Teaching Hospitals in Boston, New York, and Northern California*. Ann Arbor: University of Michigan Press, 2001.
81. Smith, Mark S., M.D., Washington, DC, by telephone 8/18/06.
82. Orlowski, Janis M., M.D., Washington, DC, by telephone 7/11/06.
83. Wartofsky, Leonard, M.D., Washington, DC, by telephone 7/20/06.
84. Drass, M. Joy, M.D., Washington, DC, by telephone 10/3/06.
85. Drass, M. Joy, M.D., Washington, DC, by e-mail 10/5/06.
86. Georgetown University Hospital/Washington Hospital Center Internal Medicine. www.whcenter.org/body.cfm?id=620. 2006.
87. McDaniel, John P., Columbia, MD, 1/13/05.

EIGHT: Georgetown University and Its Medical School

1. Corn, M. Medical Education at Georgetown. A Historical Overview. In: McFadden, WC, ed. *Georgetown at Two Hundred*. Washington, DC: Georgetown University Press, 1990, 293–319.
2. Georgetown's Catholic and Jesuit Identity. http://explore.georgetown.edu/documents/?DocumentID=736. 2006.
3. Georgetown University: a brief history. www.library.georgetown.edu/dept/speccoll/briefhis.htm. 2006.
4. Corn, Medical Education at Georgetown, 298.
5. Stapleton, JF. *Upward Journey: The Story of Internal Medicine at Georgetown 1851–1981*. Washington, DC: Georgetown University, 1996, 215.
6. Corn, Medical Education at Georgetown, 302.
7. Mitchell, Stephen Ray, M.D., Washington, DC, by telephone 7/10/06.
8. Cavender, Laura, Washington, DC, by e-mail 3/5/07.
9. McDaniel, John P., Columbia, MD, 7/13/05.

10. Bondurant, Stuart, M.D., Washington, DC, by telephone 9/7/06.

11. Goldberg, Richard L., M.D., Washington, DC, by telephone 3/23/06.

12. Drass, M. Joy, M.D., Washington, DC, 1/26/06.

13. Bloem, Kenneth D., Elk Rapids, MI, by telephone 2/20/06.

14. Bondurant, Stuart, M.D., Washington, DC, 3/28/05.

15. Mitchell, Stephen Ray, M.D., Washington, DC, by e-mail 7/18/06.

16. Haramati, Aviad, Ph.D., Baltimore, MD, 9/26/06.

17. BGRO Restructure. http://gumc.georgetown.edu/bgro—restructure.html. 2005.

18. Papadopoulos, Vassilios, Ph.D., Washington, DC, by telephone 4/10/06.

19. Morad, Martin, Ph.D., Washington, DC, by telephone 4/15/06.

20. Dimolitsas, Spiros, M.D., Washington, DC, by telephone 10/16/06.

21. Mitchell, Stephen Ray, M.D., Washington, DC, by e-mail 7/28/06.

22. Filerman, Gary L., Ph.D., Washington, DC, by telephone 3/31/06.

23. Georgetown University School of Medicine Medical Center Executive Committee 2004–2006. www3.georgetown.edu/som/faculty/facaffairs/Committees/06commit tees/ecm0406.pdf. 2006.

24. Georgetown University School of Medicine Medical Center Council of Chairs 2005–2006. www3.georgetown.edu/som/faculty/facaffairs/Committees/06committees/coc06.pdf. 2006.

25. Wiesel, Sam W., M.D., Washington, DC, by e-mail 7/18/06.

26. Siwek, Jay, M.D., Washington, DC, by telephone 8/29/06.

27. Herscowitz, Herbert B., Ph.D., Washington, DC, by telephone 9/12/06.

28. Georgetown University School of Medicine faculty tracks. file://K:/Book%20GT ,%20MedStar/GT%20faculty%20tracks.htm. 2006.

29. Herscowitz, Herbert B., Ph.D., Washington, DC, by e-mail 9/20/06.

30. Bondurant, Stuart, M.D., Washington, DC, by e-mail 1/23/07.

31. Faden, Alan I., M.D., Washington, DC, by telephone 6/14/06.

32. NIH Awards to Medical Schools by Rank. Fiscal Year 2005. http://grants.nih.gov/grants/award/rank/medttl05.htm. 2006.

33. Hawkins, Sean C., Washington, DC, by e-mail 7/5/06.

34. Lumpkin, Michael D., Ph.D., Washington, DC, 2/9/06.

35. Dretchen, Kenneth L., Ph.D., Washington, DC, 2/9/06.

36. Ford, Nelson M., Washington, DC, by telephone 4/3/06.

37. Katz, Paul, M.D., Miami, FL, by telephone 3/13/06.

38. Kim, Young, M.D., Washington, DC, by telephone 8/9/06.

39. Martuza, Robert L., M.D., Boston, MA, by telephone 7/17/06.

40. Waldhorn, Richard E., M.D., Baltimore, MD, by telephone 2/10/06.

41. Wiesel, Sam W., M.D., Washington, DC, 1/26/06.

42. Faden, Alan I., M.D., Washington, DC, by e-mail 9/25/06.

43. Davidson, Bruce J., M.D., Washington, DC, by telephone 6/15/06.

44. Goldberg, Richard L., M.D., Washington, DC, by telephone 3/15/06.

45. Lynch, John H., M.D., Washington, DC, by telephone 8/31/06.

46. Pearle, David L., M.D., Bethesda, MD, by telephone 4/4/06.

47. Pentecost, Michael J., M.D., Rockville, MD, by telephone 6/28/06.

48. Rackley, Charles E., M.D., Washington, DC, by telephone 5/24/06.

49. Schlegel, Richard, M.D., Ph.D., Washington, DC, by telephone 7/18/06.

50. Wilcox, Christopher S., M.D., Ph.D., Washington, DC, by telephone 6/14/06.

51. NIH FY 2004 Extramural Awards to Medical School Departments by NIH Department Combining Name. http://grants.nih.gov/grants/award/rank/medindp04.htm. 2005.

52. Papadopoulos, Vassilios, Ph.D., Washington, DC, by e-mail 10/10/06.

53. Dym, Martin O., Ph.D., Potomac, MD, by telephone 6/26/06.

54. Bondurant, Stuart, M.D., Washington, DC, by e-mail 3/5/07.

55. Papadopoulos, Vassilios, Ph.D., Washington, DC, by e-mail 10/9/06.

56. Morad, Martin, Ph.D., Washington, DC, by e-mail 10/17/06.

57. Clauw, Daniel J., M.D., San Diego, CA, by telephone 6/26/06.

58. Verbalis, Joseph G., M.D., Washington, DC, 1/26/06.

59. Nelson, David B., M.D., Washington, DC, by telephone 7/7/06.

60. Bloem, Kenneth D., Elk Rapids, MI, by telephone 4/13/06.

61. Anderson, Minor W., Miami, FL, by telephone 6/1/06.

62. Lippman, Marc E., M.D., Ann Arbor, MI, by telephone 3/16/06.

63. Woosley, Raymond L., M.D., Ph.D., Tucson, AZ, by telephone 4/5/06.

64. Robinowitz, Carolyn, M.D., Washington, DC, by telephone 3/5/05.

65. O'Brien, Charles M., Jr., Pittsburgh, PA, by telephone 4/7/06.

66. Pellegrino, Edmund D., M.D., Bethesda, MD, by telephone 6/23/06.

67. Rennert, Owen M., M.D., Bethesda, MD, by telephone 7/7/06.

68. Curran, Michael J., Columbia, MD, 6/6/05.

69. Cassem, Edwin H., M.D., Boston, MA, by telephone 6/3/06.

70. Lemp, Michael A., M.D., Washington, DC, by telephone 5/30/06.

71. NIH Support to U.S. Medical Schools, FY's 1970–2000. http://grants1.nih.gov/grants/award/trends/medsup7000.txt. 3/15/01.

72. Bondurant, Stuart, M.D., Washington, DC, by e-mail 6/6/06.

73. DeGioia, John J., Ph.D., Washington, DC, 11/15/06.

74. Georgetown University names Howard J. Federoff, MD, PhD, executive vice president for health sciences. http://explore.georgetown.edu/news/?ID=20935. 11/29/06.

NINE: MedStar Health

1. Merson, Michael R., Baltimore, MD, 3/5/05.

2. Thomas, William L., M.D., Columbia, MD, 6/9/05.

3. Kastor, JA. Johns Hopkins University and Hospital: Separate Governance. In: *Governance of Teaching Hospitals: Turmoil at Penn and Hopkins.* Baltimore: Johns Hopkins University Press, 2004, chap. 6, 189–193.

4. Kastor, JA. USCF Stanford: Formation. In: *Mergers of Teaching Hospitals in Boston, New York, and Northern California.* Ann Arbor: University of Michigan Press, 2001, chap. 6, 320.

5. Patricia Meisol. "Good Samaritan to Join Helix Hospital Network." *The Baltimore Sun,* 2/9/94.

6. Jay Greene. "Baltimore's Helix, Good Samaritan Set Merger Agreement." *Modern Health Care,* 3/21/94.

7. Kastor, Johns Hopkins University and Hospital, 203.

8. Merson, Michael R., Baltimore, MD, 3/9/05.

9. M. William Salganik. "Harbor's Merger into Helix Is OK'd." *The Baltimore Sun,* 11/16/95.

10. Kastor, Johns Hopkins University and Hospital, 184–185.

11. Kastor, Johns Hopkins University and Hospital, 213–277.

12. Miller, Edward D., M.D., Baltimore, MD, 4/22/05.

13. Miller, Edward D., M.D., Baltimore, MD, by e-mail 10/10/06.

14. M. William Salganik. "Helix Health's CEO Resigns. Oakey Departs amid Merger Talks. Merson Is Successor." *The Baltimore Sun*, 11/12/97.

15. M. William Salganik. "Hew Helix Chief Puts Hopkins Talks on Hold." *The Baltimore Sun*, 12/18/97.

16. John Fairhall. "Helix Health Joins the Big Leagues." *The Baltimore Sun*, 6/4/95.

17. Merson, Michael R., Baltimore, MD, 3/14/05.

18. David Segal. "Medlantic, Helix to Form Regional Hospital Network; Alliance Would Be Area's Largest and Follows Nationwide Trend." *The Washington Post*, 10/6/95.

19. Mark Guidera. "CareSystem to Base in Columbia; Helix and Medlantic Launching BWHealth in Affluent Corridor." *The Baltimore Sun*, 1/26/96.

20. Abbe Gluck. "Helix-Medlantic Venture Gets a President. Schmitt Is Given Top Post at BWHealth." *The Baltimore Sun*, 8/7/96.

21. David S. Hilzenrath. "Medlantic Healthcare, Helix Health to Merge." *The Washington Post*, 2/18/98.

22. Kastor, JA. *Mergers of Teaching Hospitals in Boston, New York, and Northern California*. Ann Arbor: University of Michigan Press, 2001.

23. M. William Salganik. "Merger of Helix, Medlantic Is Approved by Both Boards." *The Baltimore Sun*, 5/8/98.

24. McDaniel, John P., Columbia, MD, 1/13/05.

25. Kastor, Johns Hopkins University and Hospital, 189–193.

26. Curran, Michael J., Columbia, MD, by telephone 6/9/06.

27. Alan Breznick. "New Health Care Giant Begins Flexing Its Muscles; For Nonprofit Group, Challenge Is Merging Disparate Cultures." *The Washington Post*, 11/2/98.

28. M. William Salganik. "Md. Panel Names 5 CareFirst Directors." *The Baltimore Sun*, 11/22/03.

29. M. William Salganik. "CareFirst Adds 9 Reform Members to Nonprofit's Board of Directors. New Chairmen Also Are Named as Part of Shake-up by Legislature." *The Baltimore Sun*, 6/25/04.

30. Dan Thanh Dang. "Md. Lawmakers Castigate CareFirst. Implement Reform or Face Tougher Deal, Insurer Told." *The Baltimore Sun*, 6/12/03.

31. Dan Thanh Dang. "Insurance Chief Targets CareFirst Executives. Redmer Says He'll Seek Charges on 7 Violations Detailed in New Report." *The Baltimore Sun*, 7/9/03.

32. Merson, Michael R., Baltimore, MD, by e-mail 10/12/06.

33. Wyatt, Lisa M., Washington, DC, by e-mail 6/12/06.

34. Samet, Kenneth A., Columbia, MD, 7/13/05.

35. Smith, Mark S., M.D., Washington, DC, by telephone 8/18/06.

36. O'Boyle, Michael P., Cleveland, OH, by telephone 6/27/06.

37. Samet, Kenneth A., Columbia, MD, by e-mail 2/1/07.

38. Neitz, Stephen, Columbia, MD, 7/13/05.

39. Leon, Martin B., M.D., New York, NY, by telephone 8/30/05.

40. Kent, Kenneth M., M.D., Ph.D., Washington, DC.

41. Miller, Leslie W., M.D., Washington, DC, by telephone 9/18/06.

42. Wartofsky, Leonard, M.D., Washington, DC, by telephone 7/20/06.

43. Bloem, Kenneth D., Elk Rapids, MI, by telephone 2/20/06.

44. Bondurant, Stuart, M.D., Washington, DC, 3/28/05.

45. Cupples, Howard P., M.D., Annapolis, MD, by telephone 6/8/06.

46. Curran, Michael J., Columbia, MD, 6/6/05.

47. Dretchen, Kenneth L., Ph.D., Washington, DC, 2/9/06.

48. Goldberg, Richard L., M.D., Washington, DC, by telephone 3/15/06.

49. McDaniel, John P., Columbia, MD, 7/13/05.

50. Seides, Stuart F., M.D., Washington, DC, 6/29/05.

51. Verbalis, Joseph G., M.D., Washington, DC, 1/26/06.

52. Wiesel, Sam W., M.D., Washington, DC, 1/26/06.

53. Corso, Paul J., M.D., Washington, DC, by telephone 8/1/06.

54. Cassem, Edwin H., M.D., Boston, MA, by telephone 6/3/06.

55. Churchill, Winston J., J.D., Washington, DC, by telephone 10/31/06.

56. Mitchell, Stephen Ray, M.D., Washington, DC, by telephone 7/10/06.

57. Marzano, John A., Columbia, MD, by e-mail 1/25/07.

58. Howard, Barbara V., Ph.D., Washington, DC, by telephone 3/6/06.

59. NIH Support to research institutes. Fiscal year 2005. http://grants.nih.gov/grants/award/trends/resins05.htm. 2006.

60. NIH Awards to Medical Schools by Rank. Fiscal Year 2005. http://grants.nih.gov/grants/award/rank/medttl05.htm. 2006.

61. Smith, Mark S., M.D., Washington, DC, by telephone 1/25/06.

62. Ratner, Robert E., M.D., Hyattsville, MD, by e-mail 10/9/06.

63. Epstein, Stephen E., M.D., Washington, DC, by telephone 9/13/06.

64. Zager, Laurie, R.N., Washington, DC, by e-mail 10/24/06.

65. Swearingen, Christine M., Columbia, MD, by telephone 6/12/06.

66. McDaniel, John P., Columbia, MD, by e-mail 1/25/07.

TEN: Conclusions

1. Kastor, JA. Appendix 1: Governance of American Medical Centers. In: *Governance of Teaching Hospitals: Turmoil at Penn and Hopkins*. Baltimore: Johns Hopkins University Press, 2004, 295–301.

2. Blumenthal D, Weissman JS. "Selling Teaching Hospitals to Investor-owned Hospital Chains: Three Case Studies." *Health Affairs* 2000;19:158–166.

3. Williams, John F., Jr., M.D., Washington, DC, by e-mail 2/8/07.

4. Williams, John F., Jr., M.D., Washington, DC, by e-mail 10/4/06.

5. Mitchell, Stephen Ray, M.D., Washington, DC, by e-mail 9/29/06.

6. Wiesel, Sam W., M.D., Washington, DC, by telephone 10/5/06.

7. Adashi, Eli Y., M.D., Providence, RI, by e-mail 11/2/06.

8. Alpern, Robert J., M.D., New Haven, CT, by e-mail 11/1/06.

9. Antman, Karen, M.D., Boston, MA, by e-mail 11/1/06.

10. Applegate, William A., M.D., Winston-Salem, NC, by e-mail 12/14/06.

11. Bailey, David N., M.D., San Diego, CA, by e-mail 12/10/06.

12. Balke, C. William, M.D., Lexington, KY, by e-mail 11/6/06.

13. Barnes, Anne C., Oklahoma City, OK, by e-mail 12/7/06.

14. Benson, Nicholas, M.D., Greenville, NC, by e-mail 12/27/06.

15. Berk, Steven L., M.D., Lubbock, TX, by e-mail 1/3/07.

16. Boyden, Jaclyne W., New Haven, CT, by e-mail 11/3/06.
17. Buja, L. Maximillian, M.D., Houston, TX, by e-mail 11/6/06.
18. Cain, Michael E., M.D., Buffalo, NY, by e-mail 12/28/06.
19. Cesario, Thomas C., M.D., Orange, CA, by e-mail 1/3/07.
20. Cohen, Marcia J., Stanford, CA, by e-mail 11/3/06.
21. Colenda, Christopher C., M.D., College Station, TX, by telephone 11/13/06.
22. Crandall, Edward D., M.D., Ph.D., Los Angeles, CA, by telephone 11/1/06.
23. Daroff, Robert B., M.D., Cleveland, OH, by e-mail 11/3/06.
24. Deckers, Peter J., M.D., Farmington, CT, by e-mail 11/2/06.
25. Dismuke, S. Edwards, M.D., Wichita, KS, by e-mail 11/14/06.
26. Dorsey, J. Kevin, M.D., Springfield, IL, by e-mail 12/18/06.
27. Drees, Betty M., M.D., Kansas City, MO, by telephone 11/13/06.
28. Dunn, Michael J., M.D., Milwaukee, WI, by e-mail 12/15/06.
29. Enarson, Cam E., M.D., Omaha, NE, by e-mail 12/8/06.
30. Federman, Daniel D., M.D., Boston, MA, by e-mail 9/27/06.
31. Fine, Richard N., M.D., Stony Brook, NY, by e-mail 12/12/06.
32. Fiser, Debra H., M.D., Little Rock, AR, by e-mail 12/14/06.
33. Fogarty, John P., M.D., Burlington, VT, by e-mail 11/3/06.
34. Franks, Ronald D., M.D., Johnson City, TN, by e-mail 12/18/06.
35. Furnstahl, Lawrence, Chicago, IL, by e-mail 11/2/06.
36. Gabbe, Steven G., M.D., Nashville, TN, by e-mail 12/11/06.
37. Gardner, Laurence B., M.D., Miami, FL, by e-mail 12/6/06.
38. Garson, Arthur T., Jr., M.D., Charlottesville, VA, by e-mail 12/8/06.
39. Gibson, J. Scott, Durham, NC, by mail 12/14/06.
40. Golden, Robert N., Madison, WI, by e-mail 12/11/06.
41. Goldman, Lee, M.D., New York, NY, by e-mail 11/21/06.
42. Grieco, Anthony J., M.D., New York, NY, by e-mail 10/31/06.
43. Grigsby, R. Kevin, D.S.W., Hershey, PA, by e-mail 12/14/06.
44. Guzick, David S., M.D., Ph.D., Rochester, NY, by e-mail 12/8/06.
45. Halperin, Edward C., M.D., Louisville, KY, by e-mail 12/17/06.
46. Handlir, Gregory F., Baltimore, MD, by telephone 9/22/06.
47. Harris, Bradley, Columbus, OH, by e-mail 11/13/06.
48. Headrick, Linda A., M.D., Columbia, MO, by e-mail 12/20/06.
49. Henderson, Brian E., M.D., Los Angeles, CA, by e-mail 1/4/06.
50. Henrich, William L., M.D., San Antonio, TX, by e-mail 12/9/06.
51. Johns, Michael M. E., M.D., Atlanta, GA, by e-mail 10/31/06.
52. Joiner, Keith A., M.D., Tucson, AZ, by e-mail 12/14/06.
53. Kozera, Richard J., M.D., Philadelphia, PA, by e-mail 11/1/06.
54. Krane, N. Kevin, M.D., New Orleans, LA, by e-mail 11/6/06.
55. Kriech, Julie, Sioux Falls, SD, by e-mail 2/12/07.
56. Kimmel, Jennifer, M.D., Reno, NV, by e-mail 1/11/07.
57. Krugman, Richard D., M.D., Denver, CO, by e-mail 12/11/06.
58. Landsberg, Lewis, M.D., Chicago, IL, by e-mail 12/5/06.
59. LaRosa, John C., M.D., Brooklyn, NY, by e-mail 11/17/06.
60. Laughlin, Larry W., M.D., Ph.D., Bethesda, MD, by e-mail 12/8/06.
61. Lazare, Aaron, M.D., Worcester, MA, by e-mail 11/1/06.
62. Leapman, Stephen B., M.D., Indianapolis, IN, by telephone 12/14/06.
63. Levey, Gerald S., M.D., Los Angeles, CA, by e-mail 10/31/06.

64. Levine, Arthur S., M.D., Pittsburgh, PA, by e-mail 2/7/07.
65. Lieberman, Steven A., M.D., Galveston, TX, by e-mail 12/18/06.
66. Lindor, Keith D., M.D., Rochester, MN, by e-mail 11/17/06.
67. Lloyd, Sterling M., Jr., Washington, DC, by e-mail 1/5/07.
68. Lowry, Stephen F., M.D., New Brunswick, NJ, by e-mail 1/3/07.
69. McCartney, Cheryl F., M.D., Chapel Hill, NC, by e-mail 11/17/06.
70. McCloskey, Bryan L., Springfield, IL, by telephone 12/18/06.
71. Miller, D. Douglas, M.D., C.M., Augusta, GA, by e-mail 12/20/06.
72. Monteleone, Patricia L., M.D., St. Louis, MO, by e-mail 12/20/06.
73. Montgomery-Rice, Valerie, M.D., Nashville, TN, by e-mail 12/16/06.
74. Morrison, Gail, M.D., Philadelphia, PA, by telephone 10/11/06.
75. Nasca, Thomas J., M.D., Philadelphia, PA, by e-mail 10/31/06.
76. Nichols, David G., M.D., Baltimore, MD, by telephone.
77. Ostrander, Gary K., Ph.D., Honolulu, HI, by e-mail 12/16/06.
78. Peartree, Louisa A., Baltimore, MD, 9/22/06.
79. Pizzo, Philip A., M.D., Ph.D., Stanford, CA, by e-mail 11/2/06.
80. Powell, Deborah E., M.D., Ph.D., Minneapolis, MN, by e-mail 11/3/06.
81. Prescott, John E., M.D., Morgantown, WV, by e-mail 12/18/06.
82. Pyles, Brian, Toledo, OH, by telephone 12/15/06.
83. Rich, Robert R., M.D., Birmingham, AL, by e-mail 1/3/07.
84. Richardson, Mark A., M.D., Portland, OR, by e-mail 12/12/06.
85. Robillard, Jean E., M.D., Iowa City, IA, by e-mail 12/8/06.
86. Rosenblatt, Michael, M.D., Boston, MA, by e-mail 11/1/06.
87. Ross, Arthur J., III, M.D., North Chicago, IL, by e-mail 12/15/06.
88. Roth, Paul B., M.D., Albuquerque, NM, by e-mail 12/21/06.
89. Sandlow, Leslie J., M.D., Chicago, IL, by e-mail 1/2/07.
90. Sansing, Susan R., Mobile, AL, by e-mail 12/18/06.
91. Schroth, Keith, New Orleans, LA, by telephone 11/13/06.
92. Schwab, Steve J., M.D., Memphis, TN, by e-mail 1/8/07.
93. Scott, James L., Washington, DC, by telephone 11/7/06.
94. Sousa, Aron, M.D., East Lansing, MI, by e-mail 12/17/06.
95. Storey-Johnson, Carol L., M.D., New York, NY, by telephone 11/27/06.
96. Strata, Samuel, Ph.D., Mobile, AL, by e-mail 12/16/06.
97. Taylor, Robert E., M.D., Ph.D., Washington, DC, by e-mail 1/5/07.
98. Tisher, C. Craig, M.D., Gainesville, FL, by e-mail 12/15/06.
99. Werner, Leonard S., M.D., Loma Linda, CA, by e-mail 1/3/07.
100. Wesnousky, Katherine M., Davis, CA, by e-mail 12/11/06.
101. Whelton, Paul K., M.D., New Orleans, LA, by e-mail 11/6/06.
102. Wildenthal, Kern, M.D., Ph.D., Dallas, TX, by e-mail 11/28/06.
103. Wynne, Joshua, M.D., Grand Forks, ND, by e-mail 12/21/06.
104. Mount, Kenneth J., Madison, WI, by e-mail 2/1/07.
105. Schaengold, Phillip S., J.D., Syracuse, NY, by telephone 10/24/06.
106. Miller, Alan B., King of Prussia, PA, 9/19/05.
107. Judith VandeWater. "New Chief Wants to Raise Tenet's Profile in St. Louis." *St. Louis Post Dispatch*, 8/19/00.
108. Chrencik, Robert A., Baltimore, MD, by telephone 9/8/06.
109. Bass, Gerald H., Washington, DC, by telephone 11/20/06.

APPENDIX A: Other Universities with Teaching Hospitals Owned by For-Profit Companies

1. Blumenthal D, Weissman JS. "Selling Teaching Hospitals to Investor-owned Hospital Chains: Three Case Studies." *Health Affairs* 2000;19:158–166.
2. O'Brien RL, Haller MJ. "Investor-owned or Nonprofit. Issues and Implications for Academic and Ethical Values in a Catholic Teaching Hospital." *New England Journal of Medicine* 1985;313:198–201.
3. O'Brien, Richard L. Twelve years' experience with an investor-owned teaching hospital.
4. O'Brien, Richard L., M.D., Omaha, NE, by telephone 10/12/06.
5. Enarson, Cam E., M.D., Omaha, NE, by telephone 10/10/06.
6. "Tale of Two Hospitals and of Two Systems. USC Facilities Provide a Mirror of U.S. Health Care." *Modern Health Care*, 5/19/91.
7. Daniel Yi. "USC Seeks Sale of Hospital by Tenet." *Los Angeles Times*, 8/23/06.
8. Stark Law. http://en.wikipedia.org/wiki/Stark—Law, 2006
9. Rhonda L. Rundle. "USC Sues Tenet to Regain Control of Its Hospital." *Wall Street Journal*, 8/23/06.
10. Whelton, Paul K., M.D., New Orleans, LA, by telephone 10/2/06.
11. LaRosa, John C., M.D., Brooklyn, NY, by telephone 10/3/06.
12. Andrew Ross Sorkin. "HCA Buyout Highlights Era of Going Private." *The New York Times*, 7/25/06.
13. Andrews, M. Dewayne, M.D., Oklahoma City, OK, by telephone 10/10/06.
14. Judith VandeWater. "Biondi Defends Taking Tenet's Offer. Says SLU Medical School Wouldn't Have Survived." *St. Louis Post Dispatch*, 10/29/97.
15. Patricia Rice. "Tenet Seals SLU Hospital Deal. Vatican Blessed Sale of Catholic Facility for $300 Million. Jesuits Must Tighten Oversight of SLU." *St. Louis Post Dispatch*, 2/25/98.
16. Haynes, Crystal L., St. Louis, MO, by e-mail 10/18/06.
17. Mark Schlinkmann, Susan C. Thomson. "SLU Oks Sale of Hospital to For-profit firm." *St. Louis Post Dispatch*, 10/5/97.
18. Judith VandeWater. "Tenet's $300 Million Offer Ranks on the High Side." *St. Louis Post Dispatch*, 10/12/97.
19. Biondi, Lawrence H., Ph.D., St. Louis, MO, by telephone 11/1/06.
20. Di Bisceglie, Adrian M., M.D., St. Louis, MO, by telephone 10/18/06.
21. Kimmey, James R., M.D., St. Louis, MO, by telephone 10/19/06.
22. "Archbishop Won't Budge on SLU Hospital Sale. Cardinal Wonders if University Can Remain a Catholic School." *St. Louis Post Dispatch*, 10/11/97.
23. Patricia Rice, Judith VandeWater. "Leaders at SLU Aren't Buckling. They Stand by Hospital Sale despite Vatican." *St. Louis Post Dispatch*, 12/2/97.
24. Schaengold, Phillip S., J.D., Syracuse, NY, by telephone 10/24/06.
25. SLUCare. The physicians of St. Louis University. www.slucare.edu/index.php. 2006.
26. Judith VandeWater. "Hospital Workers Would Lose Free-tuition Waiver with Tenet Ownership Change. Would Also See IRA Dropped. Other Benefits Would Be Added." *St. Louis Post Dispatch*, 11/6/97.

27. Haynes, Crystal L., St. Louis, MO, by telephone 10/17/06.
28. Andrea Gerlin, Carl Stark. "Tenet Agrees to Rescue Allegheny. The Offer: $345 Million to Buy Eight Hospitals." *Philadelphia Inquirer*, 9/30/98.
29. Burns LR, Cacciamani J, Clement J, Aquino W. "The Fall of the House of AHERF: The Allegheny Bankruptcy." *Health Affairs* 2000;19:7–41.
30. Drexel University. A university with a difference. The unique vision of Anthony J. Drexel. www.drexel.edu/papadakis/newcomen/. 2001.
31. Myers, Allen R., M.D., Philadelphia, PA, by telephone 10/24/06.
32. Papadakis, Constantine, Ph.D., Philadelphia, PA, by telephone 11/21/06.
33. Linda Lloyd. "Drexel Board Backs MCP Hahnemann Deal." *Philadelphia Inquirer*, 4/26/02.
34. Papadakis, Constantine, Ph.D., Philadelphia, PA, by telephone 11/27/06.
35. Carl Stark, Josh Goldstein. "Losses Doomed MCP." *Philadelphia Inquirer*, 12/19/03.
36. Josh Goldstein. "Campus of MCP Is Sold for $11 Million. The Buyer of the East Falls Property Will Devote Space to Medical Services." *Philadelphia Inquirer*, 6/10/06.

APPENDIX B: **Reducing Deficits and Increasing Surpluses in Private Medical Schools That Do Not Own Their Primary Teaching Hospitals**

1. Adkison, Claudia R., Ph.D., Atlanta, GA, by telephone 9/7/06.
2. Barchi, Robert L., M.D., Ph.D., Philadelphia, PA, by telephone 9/25/06.
3. Black, Michael E., St. Louis, MO, by telephone 8/10/06.
4. Breault, Patrick W., Baltimore, MD, 9/11/06.
5. Carpenter, Bernard A., Baltimore, MD, by telephone 7/26/06.
6. Deeley, John M., Providence, RI, by telephone 8/1/06.
7. Elger, William R., Ann Arbor, MI, by telephone 8/14/06.
8. Ferguson, Bruce, Seattle, WA, by telephone 7/31/06.
9. Furnstahl, Lawrence, M.D., Chicago, IL, by telephone 8/28/06.
10. Gabbe, Steven G., M.D., Nashville, TN, by telephone 11/27/06.
11. Garson, Arthur T., Jr., M.D., Charlottesville, VA, by telephone 8/11/06.
12. Gibson, J. Scott, Durham, NC, by mail 9/14/06, by FAX Deficits.
13. Gilmore, Thomas N., Philadelphia, PA, by telephone 8/4/06.
14. Grossi, Richard A., Baltimore, MD, by mail 8/10/06.
15. Handlir, Gregory F., Baltimore, MD, by telephone 9/22/06.
16. Jackiewicz, Thomas E., San Diego, CA, by telephone 8/30/06.
17. Jarrell, Bruce E., M.D., Baltimore, MD, 8/3/06.
18. Marks, Lilli, Denver, CO, by telephone 8/7/06.
19. McConnell, John D., M.D., Chicago, IL, by telephone 8/1/06.
20. Miller, Jeffrey C., Chicago, IL, by telephone 8/8/06.
21. Newman, Paul, Durham, NC, by telephone 8/31/06.
22. O'Boyle, Michael P., Cleveland, OH, by telephone 7/28/06, by e-mail Deficits.
23. Peartree, Louisa A., Baltimore, MD, 8/7/06.
24. Pieper, Jay, Boston, MA, by telephone 7/25/06.
25. Rothman, Judith, Los Angeles, CA, by telephone 7/28/06.
26. Rubenstein, Arthur H., M.B., B.Ch., Philadelphia, PA, by telephone 9/12/06.
27. Schroeder, James L., M.D., Chicago, IL, by telephone 8/9/06.

28. Schwind, Ann, Chicago, IL, by telephone 9/5/06.

29. Thibault, George E., M.D., Boston, MA, by telephone 7/25/06.

30. Ziskind, Andrew A., M.D., St. Louis, MO, by e-mail 11/13/06.

31. Kastor, JA. Johns Hopkins University and Hospital: Separate Governance. In: *Governance of Teaching Hospitals: Turmoil at Penn and Hopkins*. Baltimore: Johns Hopkins University Press, 2004, chap. 6, 211–212.

32. Elger WR. "Managing Resources in a Better Way: A New Financial Management Approach for the University of Michigan Medical School." *Academic Medicine* 2006;81:301–305.

33. Miller, Edward D., M.D., Baltimore, MD, by e-mail 4/10/07.

Index

Page numbers in italics indicate illustrations in the galleries.

academic medical centers: customs of administration of, 20; financial support for, 1–2, 3; investor-owned companies and, 178–79; referral practices of, 98; in Washington, D.C., 1. *See also* Georgetown University Hospital; George Washington University Hospital
accounting systems, 195
Adkins, Mark, 37–38
administrative structure: of GWU, 72–76; of medical schools, 194–95; of MFA, 26. *See also* management
Akman, Jeffrey, 71
American Medical International, Inc., 183–84
Amsterdam, Philip, 60
aortic insufficiency, 98
Areen, Judith, 87
Aronovitch, Stanley, 47, 48
arrhythmia surgery, 99
Azumi, Norio, 123

Badger, Stephen, 26, 71
Balanced Budget Act of 1997, 3
Barch, Michael, 9, 11, 48
Barnes-Jewish Hospital, 199
basic science department (GU), 137–40
Bass, Gerald (Jerry), 24, 25, 26, 28, 30
Batshaw, Mark, 69, 70
Bayview Hospital, Baltimore, 199
benefits, 112–13, 196, 197–98
Berg, Patricia, 59
Berrigan, Michael, 30, 31–32
Betty Lou Ourisman Breast Cancer Clinic, 117
billing and collection, improving, 193–94

biomedical graduate research organization (BGRO), 131, 137, 138
biotechnology transfer, 201
Birnbaum, Philip, 34
Block, James, 152
Bloem, Kenneth, *145b;* as CEO, 88, 89; on competition, 105–6; departure of, 93; on Johns Hopkins, 90, 91; on medical center infrastructure, 85; on MedStar, 110; on university versus medical center, 83, 84, 141
Blue Cross/Blue Shield of Maryland, 147
board of trustees: GU, 81, 141; GWU, 75, 76–79; Helix, 149, 150–51, 153; MedStar Health, 157, 165–66
Bondurant, Stuart, *145a;* on candidate search, 145; on chairs of departments of medicine, 119; on clinicians, 124; Executive Committee and, 133; on firing of administrators, 137; Institute of Medicine and, 135; on Jesuits at Georgetown, 142; leadership of, 130–31, 132, 143–44; on Lombardi Cancer Center, 117; on practice plan, 125; on research, 136, 139; role of, 91; on transfers of funds, 84
Bowles, Thompson, 47
Brady, Luther, 51–52, 53, 77
Brand, Joseph, 57
Bush, George W., 15
business plans, 200
BWHealth, 154–55

Campbell, Karen, 119, 120
capital programs of hospitals, 201
Carbonell, Nelson, 78–79
cardiology and cardiac surgery: consolidation of, 125–26; at GUH, 97–103; at GWUH, 35–39; at Washington Hospital Center, 160–61

Cardiovascular Research Institute, 168
CareFirst, Blue Cross/Blue Shield, 158
Carroll, John, 128
Cassem, Edwin (Ned), 142, 143, *145b*, 164
Cavender, Laura, 92
census, average daily: GUH, 94; GWUH, 6, 18;
   Washington Hospital Center, 159
centralized system for billing and collection,
   193–94
Cerqueira, Manuel, 99
certificate of need. *See* CON
chairmen of clinical departments: GU, 119–
   24, 137–38; GWU, 20, 32–34; proposals between hospital director and, 201; recruitment of, 175–77
Chapman, Thomas, 2, 3, 8, 14, 54
Cheney, Dick, 15
chiefs of service, 20–21
Children's National Medical Center, 69–70,
   101–2, 159
Church Hospital and Home, Baltimore, 151–
   52
Churchill, Winston, 164
Clauw, Daniel, 139
clinical education, financial support for, 110,
   118, 174–75
clinical educator track, 134
"clinical" in academic title, 37
clinician scholar track, 134
clinician track, 134
clinics (GWU), 44–45
co-chair system, 122–23
Cohen, Sheldon, 8
Columbian College, 49, 50
Community Practice Network, 106
CON (certificate of need), 11, 16–17
consultants, using, 202–3
Corcoran, William Wilson, 50
Corn, Milton: as dean, 81, 82; on Griffith, 86–
   87; on history of GU, 128, 129; on Lippman,
   116; resignation of, 83
Corso, Paul, 101, 102, 164
Cosgrove, Delos, 9
Cossman, Jeffrey, 117
Council of Chairs, 133
Cox, James, 99–100
Creighton University, 143, 183–84

Cullen, Kevin, 117
Cupples, Howard, 118–19
Curran, Mike, 165
Curzon, Myron, 78

dean, powers of, 124–25
dean's tax, 27, 84, 194
debt/endowment ratio, 90
debt to university, 198
deficit-producing units, solutions for, 197
deficits, growth and, 202
DeGioia, John, *145a*; Bondurant and, 91; on
   candidate search, 145; on practice plan, 110;
   as president, 140–41; role of, 87; tenure
   buyout and, 111, 112
dental school, closing of, 85
diagnosis-related group (DRG) system and
   GWUH, 7
Dimolitsas, Spiros, 132
dispensary, 51
District of Columbia General Hospital, 7, 159–60
District Partners, LLP, 13
divestment: of GUH, 89–97; of GWUH, 6–10
downstream revenue, 40
Drass, Joy, *145b*; on cardiac program, 100; criticism of, 96–97; emergency medicine and,
   125; Executive Committee and, 133; P. Katz
   and, 120–21; Meador on, 122; pediatric cardiac program and, 101–2; Pentecost and,
   123; practice plan and, 109, 110, 115; as
   president, 93–94; salaries and, 124; Wartofsky and, 126
Dretchen, Kenneth, 139–40
Drexel University, 190–91
DRG. *See* diagnosis-related group
Dritschilo, Anatoly, 132
Dym, Martin, 137

earnings before interest, taxes, and depreciation (EBITD), 178
Eisenberg, John, 107, 119–20
El-Bayoumi, Jehan, 71
electrophysiology laboratory, 102
Elliott, Lloyd, 34, 72, 73, 76–77
emergency department: assignment of patients from, 39; GWUH, 6, 9; merged, 125;
   visits per year, 105

endowment: debt/endowment ratio, 90; GU, 89; GU pharmacology department, 140; GWUH, 76–77, 78; GWU medical school, 62; increasing, 201; operating losses and, 202

Epstein, Stephen, 168

Epstein, Steven, 113, 114

Eugene Meyer Pavilion, 52

Evans, Stephen, 104–5, 115

Executive Committee, 133

expenses, reducing, 195–98

facilities: building new, 16–19, 146–47; GUH, investment in, 96; GWUH, description of, 6–7, 22; of MedStar Health, 92; of Universal Health Services, Inc., 15

faculty: financial issues and, 192; GUH voluntary, 95–96, 99, 108–9; GWUH voluntary, 34–42; incentives for, 201–2; tracks of, at GU, 133–35; Universal Health Services, Inc., 21–22; Washington Hospital Center voluntary, 160. *See also* Faculty Physician Group; Medical Faculty Associates, Inc.; practice plans; recruitment issues; salary issues; tenure issues

Faculty Physician Group (FPG): development of, 108–10; surplus of, 109; takeover of by MedStar, 110–15

Faden, Alan: on financial issues, 87; Griffith and, 82; on leadership, 144; on MedStar, 96, 97; on research, 135, 136

Fairfax Hospital, 71, 91, 119, 161

family medicine, department of, 106

Faselis, Charles, 64

Federoff, Howard J., 145, 176, 181

fellowships, 119, 126

Filerman, Gary, 141

financial issues: faculty and, 192; Faden on, 87; GWU medical school and, 59; MedStar Health and, 168; Washington Hospital Center and, 159–60. *See also* losses, financial

financial support: for academic medical centers, 1–2, 3; for academic mission, 180–81; for clinical education, 110, 118, 174–75; for GWUH, 7, 52; for GWU medical school, 62; MedStar, GU, and, 94; for MFA, 31; of voluntary faculty, 39–40

fiscal affairs advisory committee, 194–95

Flexner Report: GU medical school and, 129; GWU medical school and, 51

Foggy Bottom, 52

Ford, Nelson, 87

for-profit hospital-owning companies: GUH and, 91; GWUH and, 11; teaching hospitals and, 178–79, 183–91. *See also* Universal Health Services, Inc.

Fox, Harold, 55

FPG. *See* Faculty Physician Group

Franklin Square Hospital, Baltimore: Emergency Physician group and, 125; history of, 146–48; merger with Union Memorial Hospital, 148–50, 151

fundraising, 77–79, 115, 142–43. *See also* endowment

Garcia, Jorge, 98

Georgetown Practice Group, 110, 117–19

Georgetown University (GU): GUH and, 83–84; history of, 128–30; medical center and, 140–41

Georgetown University Hospital (GUH), *145a;* cardiology and cardiac surgery at, 97–103; Catholic nature of, 127; clinics of, 105–7; financial problems of, 85–87; finding buyer for, 89–93; geographical problems of, 105; governance of, 81–83; GU and, 83–84; history of, 130; losses of, 80–81; MedStar and, 93–97, 161–64; primary care clinics, 106–7; selling of, 89–97; surgery at, 103–5; Washington Hospital Center and, 119, 125–27; Wiesel and, 87–89. *See also* Faculty Physician Group

Georgetown University Law School, 87

Georgetown University Medical Center. *See* medical schools (GU)

George Washington University (GWU), administration of, 72–76

George Washington University Hospital (GWUH), *79a;* divestment of, 6–10; faculty and, 21–22; founding of, 51–53; McLean and, 19–21; new building for, 16–19, *79a;* selling of, 10–14; Universal Health Services, Inc., and, 13–16. *See also* Medical Faculty Associates, Inc.

George Washington University School of Medicine. *See* medical schools (GWU)

Gersh, Bernard, 99, 102

Ghezzi, Keith, 8, 56

Giordano, Joseph, 30, 37, 38

Goldberg, Richard: as chief medical officer, 114; on MedStar bid, 92; practice plan and, 110; salaries and, 124; on takeover of practice plan, 113, 117; on Wiesel and Bloem, 88

Goldstein, Allan, 62–63, 65

Good Samaritan Hospital, Baltimore, 150–51, 153

governance: of GUH, 81–83; of GU medical center, 132–33

Grant, U. S., III, 52

grants: Children's National Medical Center and, 69; GWU faculty and, 27; GWU medical school and, 60–61; investigators with, recruitment of, 65; MedStar Research Institute, 167; salary and, 139, 201

Greenberg, Warren, 3

Griffith, John: closing of dental school and, 85; departure of, 86–87; Eisenberg and, 120; as executive vice president, 81–83; faculty and, 95–96, 108; on financial losses, 80; Kent and, 100; Morad and, 138, 139; primary care and, 106–7; sale of hospital and, 90; tenure expense and, 86; Wallace and, 103

growth, and deficits, 202

GU. *See* Georgetown University

GUH. *See* Georgetown University Hospital

Gurne, Patricia, 10–11, 77

GWU. *See* George Washington University

GWUH. *See* George Washington University Hospital

Harbor Hospital, Baltimore, 152

Harvey, W. Proctor, 97, 98

HCA (Hospital Corporation of America), 185–87

Health Services Cost Review Commission, 147, 152

Healton, Edward, 115, 127

Healy, Timothy, 82, 83–84, 107, 142

Helix: Church Hospital and Home and, 151–52; founding of, 149–50; Good Samaritan

Hospital and, 150–51; Harbor Hospital and, 152; Johns Hopkins Hospital and, 152–54; Medlantic Healthcare Group merger with, 154–57

Heyssel, Robert, 152

Hirshfield, Anne, 66

HMO: Franklin Square and, 147; GWU, 44–48; transfers from hospital to, 8

Hochberg, Mark, 75

Hotez, Peter, 68–69

Howard, Barbara, 167

Howard University, 2

Hufnagel, Charles, 97, 98

Human Hookworm Vaccine Initiative, 68

Hunter Group, 47

income, increasing, 199–201

Inova Health System, 91

intensive care unit (GWUH), 18

interviewees, 204–31

interview methods, ix

investigators: Georgetown versus Hospital Center, 167; with grants, recruitment of, 65

Jacobson, Robert, 107

Jarrett, Thomas, 33, 66

Jesuit leadership of Georgetown University, 142–43

Johns Hopkins Hospital, 2, 4, 150, 152–54, 199

Johns Hopkins Medicine, 90–91

Kastor, Elizabeth, ix

Katz, Louis: on closing medical school, 25; Meyer and, 54–55, 56; on MFA, 23; on practice plan, 43; on reserve, 28; on selling HMO, 48; on selling hospital, 10

Katz, Nevin, 37, 111

Katz, Paul, 89, 120, 137

Katz, Richard, 35, 36, 39

Kayser, Elmer Louis, 49

Kelly, John, 32, 66, 67

Kelly, Michael, 87, 114

Keltner, Bette, 132

Kent, Kenneth, 100, 160

Knapp, Steven, 79, 179

laboratory space, 65, 68, 178, 198
LaRosa, John, 4
Lazarus, Gerald, 61, 62, 63, 77
Lehman, Donald, 32
Leon, Martin, 160
Lincoln, Abraham, 159
Lippman, Marc, 115, 116–17
Lombardi, Vince, 115–16
Lombardi Comprehensive Cancer Center,
    115–17, 123, 131, 132
Loop, Floyd, 9
losses, financial: endowment and, 202; GUH,
    80–81, 88–89, 99–100, 163; GU medical
    school, 92; GWUH, 5, 7–8, 10; to GWU
    HMO, 46, 47, 48; GWU medical center, 58;
    MFA, 24, 25, 30; overview of, ix; sale of hos-
    pitals and, 171–72; sustainability and, 192;
    Trachtenberg and, 75; Union Memorial Hos-
    pital, 149
Lough, Frederick, 38–39
Loyola-Stritch University, 143
Lumpkin, Michael, 137–38
Lustbader, Jay, 119

malpractice insurance, 169, 197
malpractice trust, 27–28
managed care, and practice plans, 194
management: of academic departments, 123–
    24; of academic medical centers, 20; of GUH
    by MedStar, 93–97; of GWU, 72–76; of
    GWU medical school, 56–60, 66–68; of
    medical schools, 194–95; by MedStar, com-
    pared to GU, 95; of MedStar, 157–58, 164–
    66; of practice plan, 24
Manatt, Charles, 10, 58, 77, *79b*
Martin, Cloyd Heck, 72
Martuza, Robert, 97, 117
Marzano, John, 165
Maxted, William, 82
Mayo Clinic, 103
McAllen Medical Center, 20
McDaniel, John, *170a;* cardiac program and,
    101; GUH and, 96, 161–62, 163, 164; on
    health care, 157; MedStar Health and, 157–
    58, 164; Merson and, 154; resignation of,
    170; Washington Hospital Center and, 165
McLean, Daniel: as CEO, 19–21; on emergency

department, 6; on neighborhood relations,
    17; on on-call rooms, 22; on practice plan,
    43; on voluntary faculty, 35
Meador, Kimford, 96–97, 121–22
Medicaid, 2, 3
"medical arms race," 18, 156
medical educator track, 134–35
Medical Faculty Associates, Inc. (MFA): ap-
    pointment of chairmen, 32–34; complaints
    of faculty, 26–29; costs to medical center of,
    58; criticism of, 42; HMO and, 47; malprac-
    tice trust and, 27–28; operations and fi-
    nances of, 29–31, 173; praise for, 43;
    proposal for, 23–25; research, education,
    and, 31–32, 65, 180; right of "first refusal"
    and, 38; Scott and, 59–60; structure of, 26;
    voluntary faculty and, 40–42
medical schools: administrative structure of,
    194–95; financial issues in, 192; incentives,
    201–2; increasing income of, 199–201;
    Jesuit, and research support, 143; reducing
    expenses of, 195–98; relationship to practice
    plans, 193–94; transfers of funds from, 8–9,
    84. *See also* medical schools (GU); medical
    schools (GWU)
medical schools (GU): basic science depart-
    ment, 137–40; chairmen of clinical depart-
    ments, 119–24; dean, powers of, 124–25;
    education at, 117–19; faculty tracks, 133–
    35; future of, 180–81; governance of, 132–
    33; history of, 128–30; Jesuit influence and,
    142–43; research at, 131–32, 135–36; re-
    structuring of, 130–32; university and, 140–
    41
medical schools (GWU): administration of,
    56–60, 66–68; chairmen of clinical depart-
    ments, 20, 32–34; communication network,
    66–67; divestment of, 5–6; education at, 70–
    72; establishment and history of, 49–51; fi-
    nancial obligations of, 59; future of, 179–80;
    research and, 60–69; Trachtenberg and, 74–
    76; Vice President for Medical Affairs posi-
    tion, 53–56; Washington Hospital Center
    and, 161
medicine, chairmen of department of, 119–21,
    122–23
Medlantic Healthcare Group: Helix merger

Medlantic Healthcare Group (*cont.*)
with, 154–57; history of, 159; lobbying campaign by, 11–12; sale to Universal and, 14; Washington Hospital Center and, 12
MedStar Health: administration of, 164–66; benefits paid by, 112–13; board of trustees of, 157; chairmen of clinical departments and, 122, 123; criticisms of, 125; executive vice president for medical affairs, 166; facilities of, 92; features of, 156–57; financial status of, 168; future of, 181; GUH and, 161–64; history of, 156; management of GUH by, 93–97; officers of, 157–58; plans of, 168–70; practice plan and, 109, 110–15, 174; primary care clinics and, 107; research and, 136. *See also* Drass, Joy
MedStar Research Institute, 167
Merson, Michael: BWHealth and, 154–55; as CEO, 147; Helix and, 148, 149, 150–51, 152, 153–54; MedStar Health and, 156–58
Meyer, Roger, 36, 54–56
MFA. *See* Medical Faculty Associates, Inc.
military hospitals, 2. *See also specific hospitals*
Miller, Alan, 14–15, 16, *79a*, 105, 178
Miller, Edward, 90–91, 153, 199
Miller, Leslie, 103, 126
Mitchell, Ray, 101, 117–18, 131, 132, 133
Monroe, James, 49
Morad, Martin, 101, 132, 138–39
Mrazek, David, 21

Najam, Farzad, 38, 39
National Institutes of Health (NIH): Children's National Medical Center and, 69; collaboration with, 3–4; GU basic science departments and, 137; GU medical center and, 135, 143; GWU department of medicine and, 32, 60–61; GWU HMO and, 45; Lombardi Cancer Center and, 116; MFA and, 31
National Medical Enterprises, 184–85
National Naval Medical Center, 2
National Rehabilitation Hospital, 159
Nauta, Russell, 103
neurology, chairmen of department of, 121–22
NIH. *See* National Institutes of Health

Oakey, James, 150–51, 153–54, 155
O'Boyle, Michael, 88, 163
O'Brien, Charles, 82, 83, 84, 100
O'Donovan, Leo, 87, 88, 93, 107
O'Leary, Dennis, 9, 34–35
on-call rooms (GWUH), 22
operating costs (GWUH), 9
operating margins (GWUH), 19
operating rooms (GWUH), 22
ophthalmology, department of, 118–19
Orlowski, Janis, 127
OrnDa HealthCorp, 12
Ott, John, 45, 46, 48
outpatient clinic (GWU), 51, 52
overhead, 198, 202
overhead recovery rate, 201

pancreatic resections, 104
Papadopoulos, Vassilios, 131, 132, 138
Pawlson, Gregory, 44, 48
payments to university, 198. *See also* dean's tax
Pearle, David, 104
Pellegrino, Edmund, 83
Pentecost, Michael, 96, 102, 111, 115, 123
Perry, Robert, 10, 43, 78
Pestell, Richard, 117
pharmacology department, 139–40
philanthropy, 77–79, 115, 142–43
PHN. *See* Preferred Health Network
physical diagnosis, 97–98
Piemme, Thomas, 44, 45
population of Washington, D.C., 2, 3
Potter, John, 116
PPO. *See* preferred provider organization
practice plans: Children's National Medical Center, 69; complaints of faculty about, 25, 26–29; MedStar-owned, 169; problems with and solutions for, 193–94; recruitment issues and, 175–77; sale of, 172–74; transfers from hospital to, 8–9. *See also* Faculty Physician Group; Medical Faculty Associates, Inc.
Preferred Health Network (PHN), 147, 148
preferred provider organization (PPO), 147
Price, Luther, 49
Price Jones, Laurel, 77
primary care clinics: GUH, 106–7; GWUH, 58
Prince George's Hospital Center, 7

private practice, MedStar and, 169
Providence Hospital, 106
purchasing, 198

Ratner, Robert, 167–68
Reagan, Ronald, 9, 15
receivership, 197
recruitment issues: GU medical center, 136,
    138, 140; and investigators with own grants,
    65; overview of, 175–77
Reiss, David, 21, 32, 60, 67–68
Rennert, Owen, 118–19
research: Children's National Medical Center
    and, 69–70; GU medical center and, 131–32,
    135–36, 180; GWU medical school and, 31,
    60–69, 179–80; history of GWU and, 53;
    Jesuit medical schools and, 143; at Lombardi
    Cancer Center, 117; MedStar Research In-
    stitute, 167; MFA and, 31–32; overview of,
    177–78
research track, 135
residencies, 126
Retchin, Sheldon, 48
Rickles, Frederick, 65–66
Rogers, Mark, 6
Rosenberg, Joel, 36–37, 40
Ross Hall, 52, 53

salary issues: grants and, 139, 201; GU practice
    plan and, 124; GWU practice plan and, 25;
    incentive plan, 109; mission-based compen-
    sation, 195–97; Reiss and, 67–68; tenure
    and, 86
Samet, Kenneth, *170a;* on boards of trustees,
    166; on cardiac program, 101; on Drass, 94;
    future of, 170; GUH and, 163; Washington
    Hospital Center and, 159, 160, 165
Schaengold, Phillip, 2, 8, 15–17, 178–79
Schimpff, Stephen, 35, 53–54
Schlegel, Richard, 123
Scott, James, 33, 59–60, 62, 77, *79b*
Sedmak, Daniel, 143
Seides, Stuart, 97
Sekhar, Laligam, 56
selling hospitals: financial losses and, 171–72;
    GUH, 89–97; GWUH, 10–14
Seneff, Michael, 19

Shalala, Donna, 74
Shesser, Robert, 9
Sibley Hospital, 161
Silber, John, 72, 74
Silva, Carlos, 39, 41–42
Simon, David, 42
Singleton, Knox, 91
Siwek, Jay, 106, 114
Smith, Mark, 6, 125, 127, 167
Solomon, Allen, 102
space issues, 198. *See also* laboratory space
spending, unbudgeted, 197
Spies, James, 118
St. Louis Children's Hospital, 199
St. Louis University, 143, 187–89
St. Louis University Hospital, 13
Stanford University hospital, 149
Stapleton, John, 119, 129
students: money spent on clinical instruction
    for, 174–75; quality of, 63, 117–18
surpluses, 202
Swearingen, Christine, 169, 170

teaching, clinical, money for, 174–75
teaching hospitals: medical schools in deficit
    and, 200; owned by for-profit companies,
    183–91
telephone costs, 198
Tenet Healthcare, 12–13, 187–91
tenure issues: GU medical center, 138; MedStar
    and, 111, 113; Reiss and, 67; at retirement,
    GU and, 86
tenure track, 134
Thomas, William: Executive Committee and,
    133; on Franklin Square Hospital merger
    with Union Memorial Hospital, 148–49;
    GUH and, 164; role of, 127, 166, 167
Trachtenberg, Stephen Joel, *79b;* on education,
    71; fundraising and, 77–78; on medical
    school, 5–6; Medlantic and, 12; Meyer and,
    54–55; practice plan and, 25, 29; as presi-
    dent, 72–76; replacement plan and, 9; on re-
    search, 61; sale of hospital and, 10; Schimpff
    on, 53, 54; on transfers from law school, 8;
    J. Williams and, 57
Tracy, Cynthia, 102
transfers of funds: from medical schools, 8–9,

transfers of funds (*cont.*)
84; to medical schools, 199; to university,
198. *See also* dean's tax
transparency in school-hospital relationship,
199–200
Tulane University, 185–86

Union Memorial Hospital, Baltimore: culture
of, 151; Emergency Physician group and,
125; merger with Franklin Square Hospital,
148–50
Universal Health Services, Inc.: facilities of, 15;
faculty conflict with, 21–22; improvements
made by, 16–19; opinions about, 18–19;
purchase of GWUH by, 13–16; research and,
179–80
University of California, San Francisco, hospital, 149
University of Oklahoma, 186–87
University of Southern California, 184–85

"veil of secrecy" at GWUH, 13
Verbalis, Joseph, 96, 121, 122, 123
Veterans Affairs Medical Center, 64, 71, 159
Virginia, patients from, 2–3
voluntary faculty: at GUH, 95–96, 99, 108–9;
at GWUH, 34–42; at Washington Hospital
Center, 160

Waldhorn, Richard, 121, 123–24
Wallace, Robert, 103–4
Walsh, Raymond, 63
Walter Reed Army Medical Center, 2
Wartofsky, Leonard, 126, 127, 169
Washington, D.C.: academic medical centers
in, 1; environment of, 2–4; Foggy Bottom,
52; medical practice in, 4

Washington Hospital Center, *170a;* affiliation
with GUH, 119; campus of, 159; cardiac program of, 35, 100, 101, 103, 160–61; Chapman on, 3; Children's National Medical
Center and, 70; consolidation of programs
with GUH, 125–27; DRGs and, 7; financial
status of, 159–60; GWU medical school and,
161; helicopter service, 160; history of, 158–
59; Medlantic and, 12; MedStar Health and,
92
Washington Institute of Thoracic and Cardiovascular Surgery, 37
Washington University, 199
Wasserman, Alan, *79b;* on chairmen, 33;
MFA and, 23, 24, 26; on salaries, 25, 30; on
J. Williams, 56–57
Weglicki, William, 64, 65
Weingold, Allan, 13, 15, 19, 28, 55
Wiesel, Sam, *145b;* on combining GWUH and
GUH, 105; Council of Chairs and, 133; Cox
and, 99–100; as executive vice president,
87–89; Johns Hopkins and, 90; P. Katz and,
120, 121; role of, 82; takeover of practice
plan and, 113–15
Williams, Edward Bennett, 116
Williams, John, Jr. (Skip), *79a;* on board, 77;
criticism of, 59; faculty and, 21; gay issues
and, 71; on history of medical school, 53;
malpractice trust and, 28; on MFA, 24–25;
on old GWU hospital, 6–7; on practice plan,
43; on research, 32; on Universal ownership,
19; as vice president, 56–58, 59–60; on voluntary faculty, 40
Woosley, Raymond, 140

Zeglis, John, 7